SOCIAL DETERMINANTS OF HEALTH TOOLKIT

Maximizing Your SDOH Scores for Stronger Community Impact, Improved Patient Outcomes, and Sustainable Health Equity – Even if You're Unsure Where to Start

Dr. Jeremy Holloway

Edited by Ryan Dale

Formatting by Muhammad Najib Ullah

INTRODUCTION

Maria never imagined that her zip code would matter more to her health than her doctor's advice. Yet every time she missed a medical appointment because the clinic was too far away, or chose fast food because fresh groceries were out of reach, the reality became clear: health isn't just about personal choices—it's about opportunities. Opportunities to access care, eat well, feel safe, and build a life not defined by barriers.

Consider a world where everyone has equal access to resources that promote health and well-being. In that world, no one has to wonder if they can afford both a healthy meal and a bus ticket to work. This may sound idealistic, but it is achievable. The Social Determinants of Health (SDOH) are at the heart of this possibility. These factors—our environment, education, income, and social connections—are not abstract concepts; they shape how our lives unfold every day.

Think of James, a young father working two jobs to support his family. Despite his determination, his neighborhood lacks safe spaces for his children to play, the closest grocery store is miles away, and his work schedule leaves little room for preventive healthcare visits. James isn't asking for pity; he's looking for a chance. Stories like James's are everywhere, and they show how communities either thrive or struggle based on these wider factors.

This toolkit is grounded in such real stories, offering tools and strategies to change outcomes for people like James—and for you.

Who is this book for? It's for individuals who want to thrive and move past mere survival. It's for caregivers striving to create better lives for their loved ones. It's for healthcare professionals, educators, and community leaders who see these challenges and want to make a difference. If you've ever felt frustrated by the inequities you witness or experience, this book offers a path forward. You don't need all the answers—you just need the willingness to act.

Why now? Because understanding and addressing SDOH is urgent. Our interconnected world has magnified disparities, but it has also given us tools to address them. This book isn't about lofty ideals or theoretical models; it's about actionable insights you can apply to your life, community, or organization.

What will you gain from this toolkit? You will:

- Discover where you currently stand in terms of SDOH and identify key areas for improvement.
- Learn practical, proven strategies to enhance these areas and create meaningful change.
- Gain tools to support others—whether as a caregiver, professional, or advocate—in overcoming barriers.
- Be inspired by stories of resilience and innovation that show what's possible when we address SDOH with intention.

The structure of this book will guide you step by step. In the opening sections, we delve into the core elements of SDOH and how they impact everyday life. From there, you'll explore practical tools and strategies for addressing these determinants. We close with stories, exercises, and plans that bring everything together, showing how even small changes can lead to significant improvements.

This toolkit is your companion in building a life—and a world—that truly thrives. This process begins with understanding, but it doesn't stop there. Together, we can take the steps needed to reshape opportunities and create brighter futures for everyone.

SECTION 1

FOUNDATIONS OF SOCIAL DETERMINANTS OF HEALTH

One day, a man was walking through his neighborhood, enjoying the first days of summer. The air was warm, the birds were singing, and flowers along the path were starting to bloom. As he strolled, he noticed a neighbor gardening in a very puzzling way. The neighbor was crouched over each plant, carefully uprooting it and pouring water directly onto its bare roots.

Curious and slightly concerned, the man approached the gardener and asked, "What are you doing?"

Without looking up, the gardener replied, "I'm watering my plants so they get all the nutrients they need. I like to get as close as I can and make sure the water has direct contact with the roots, because I know how much plants need water—especially the roots."

The man stood there for a moment, then said gently, "I think the best way to make sure the plant thrives is to keep it planted in its soil."

The gardener paused, looked at the man, and slowly nodded. He began gently placing the plants back into the soil.

This simple story highlights a truth about human life as well. Just as plants are meant to stay rooted in soil that provides nutrients, stability, and a foundation to thrive, we too need to remain connected to the "soil" of our lives: our social environments. Our social connections, our communities, and the broader circumstances of our lives create the foundation for our psychological, social, and even physical well-being.

From infancy to older adulthood, staying rooted in supportive and nurturing environments is critical. When those roots are disturbed—whether through disconnection, inequity, or lack of resources—we create less-than-ideal conditions for growth, health, and fulfillment.

This is where the Social Determinants of Health come into focus. They represent the areas in which we can observe and nurture our "roots" to ensure we remain connected and healthy. SDOH encompass factors like education, access to healthcare, neighborhood and physical environment, economic stability, and social relationships. These determinants don't just influence individual well-being—they form the foundation of thriving communities and societies.

As we explore the foundations of SDOH, consider this: Are your roots firmly planted in the soil of social connection and opportunity? If not, how can we identify and address the gaps? Together, we will unpack how these factors shape our health and explore the potential for growth in our communities and beyond.

In many fields—particularly healthcare and public health—significant resources are allocated toward managing symptoms and conducting biomedical research rather than addressing the root causes of health decline (such as social isolation and lack of purpose). This raises an important question: Are we trying to sustain a plant that has been removed from its nourishing soil, rather than restoring it to the soil it needs? In other words, when people are socially disconnected or living without a sense of purpose, is the real solution to "replant" them into a supportive community?

Disconnection and Decline

Human beings, much like plants, require a nourishing environment to thrive. Research shows that social connections and a sense of purpose act as essential "soil" for mental and physical well-being. When individuals are removed from this soil—whether through social isolation, lack of meaningful engagement, or societal structures that devalue certain groups—they often experience declines in health that mirror a plant wilting without nutrients.

Current studies on healthcare funding reveal a tendency to treat the symptoms of disease—akin to examining the roots of a plant while ignoring the soil that sustains it. In doing so, the core issues of disconnection and purposelessness can remain unaddressed, undermining efforts to improve long-term outcomes. Without recognizing that individuals need to be "replanted" into their communities, policies and interventions may fail to achieve sustained health improvements.

The Soil of Social Connection: Evidence suggests that increasing social engagement and meaningful activities can prevent or slow cognitive decline and improve mental health. This aligns with the idea that people, like plants, cannot thrive in isolation. Studies have shown that interventions designed to enhance social connections—particularly among older adults—yield positive results in health outcomes and even reduce healthcare costs.

A Call for Change: To achieve meaningful progress in public health, we must shift focus from merely treating symptoms to addressing underlying causes of decline. Our work has found that while clinical interventions play a role, policy changes that promote social inclusion and purposeful living are even more important. If we truly seek to restore health and well-being, we must recognize that individuals need to be "plugged back into the soil where they belong." Efforts should be directed toward rebuilding the social connections that are vital to sustaining human health. That is what we aim to do in this toolkit.

In short: Are we spending resources trying to keep a plant alive outside of its soil, when we should be restoring it to nourishing ground? In human terms, treating medical issues without addressing social disconnection is unlikely to lead to lasting health. Real health improvements require re-connecting people to supportive communities and environments.

Key Point: Put the plant back in the soil. In human terms, ensure people are connected to supportive social environments if you want them to thrive.

Our Journey Back to the Soil

Treating roots without returning the plant to nourishing soil may create a superficial form of health rather than an authentic recovery. Similarly, addressing human health requires more than medical treatments—it demands reconnection to a supportive social environment that nourishes purpose and engagement. The plant-and-soil metaphor serves as a reminder that effective health interventions should prioritize a holistic approach, emphasizing social integration as a critical component of care.

What Are SDOH? Social Determinants of Health are the conditions in which we are born, grow, live, work, and age. They are the social, economic, and environmental factors that shape our health and well-being more than we often realize. While healthcare and personal choices are crucial, SDOH represent the "soil" in which our health and potential are rooted. Just as a plant's health depends on the quality of its soil, our well-being is deeply influenced by the environments we navigate every day.

SDOH can be categorized into five key areas as defined by public health experts: **Economic Stability, Education Access and Quality, Healthcare Access and Quality, Neighborhood and Built Environment, and Social and Community Context.** We have also added two additional areas that play significant roles: Food and Nutrition and Work and Recreation—making seven determinants in total. Each category is interconnected, forming a complex web of influence over our lives. Let's explore each of these in depth and understand their profound impact on health and well-being.

- **Economic Stability:** This is about having the financial resources to afford housing, food, healthcare, and other essentials. Financial security reduces stress and provides stability that promotes mental and physical health. Example: Sarah, a single mother juggling two jobs, often must choose between buying groceries and paying the electric bill. The chronic stress of living paycheck to paycheck takes a toll on her health, increasing her risk for high blood pressure and diabetes. Limited income also makes it hard to afford fresh, nutritious food, leaving her family reliant on cheaper processed options that lack nutrients. For someone like Sarah, improving economic stability—through higher income, job training, or financial assistance—would lay a practical foundation for overall well-being. Without economic stability, individuals are constantly uprooted by the struggle to meet basic needs.

- **Education Access and Quality:** Education is a key determinant of opportunity, influencing health literacy, employment prospects, and the ability to advocate for oneself and one's family. Access to quality education is like planting seeds in fertile ground—when nurtured, those seeds grow into strong, resilient plants capable of weathering life's challenges. Disparities in education can create long-term inequities. Example: Children in underfunded schools may lack access to experienced teachers and advanced coursework, putting them at a disadvantage early in life. On the other hand, education empowers individuals: someone who is well-educated is more likely to secure stable employment, understand medical information, and make informed health decisions. Ensuring equitable access to quality education means communities have the tools to thrive, not just survive.
- **Healthcare Access and Quality:** Healthcare is often viewed as the primary driver of health outcomes, but simply having access to care isn't enough. The quality of care, its cultural relevance, and its physical accessibility are all critical. Example: Carlos finally gets health insurance through his job—an important step forward—but the nearest clinic is a 45-minute

drive away, and he struggles to get time off work for appointments. When he does see a doctor, the providers seem rushed and no one speaks his primary language, which creates barriers to understanding his treatment plan. Healthcare should be like water reaching the roots of a plant—not merely available, but also nourishing and effective. Improving healthcare access means not only having services available, but ensuring those services are affordable, culturally sensitive, and delivered in a patient-centered way.

- **Neighborhood and Built Environment:** The physical spaces we live in profoundly impact our health and quality of life. Safe housing, reliable transportation, access to green spaces, clean air, and nearby grocery stores all contribute to well-being. Example: Mia is a teenager in a densely populated urban area. Her small, poorly ventilated apartment worsens her asthma. The nearest park is miles away, limiting her ability to play and exercise. Unreliable public transport makes doctor visits stressful and time-consuming. By contrast, a community with clean air, accessible parks, and safe housing provides fertile soil for residents to thrive. Neglected neighborhoods can harm health and reinforce cycles of inequity. Addressing this means improving housing conditions, infrastructure, and environmental safety so that where you live doesn't determine how healthy you can be.
- **Social and Community Context:** Human beings are inherently social. Our relationships with family, friends, coworkers, and neighbors provide support, a sense of belonging, and purpose. These connections

are like roots that anchor us during life's storms. Example: Daniel is an older adult living alone after his spouse's passing. With very little social interaction, his sense of isolation grows, leading to increased stress and declining health. Meanwhile, his neighbor Lily stays active at a community center, participating in group activities that keep her socially and mentally engaged. Lily's community support buffers her against loneliness and poor health. Belonging is more than a feeling—it's a protective factor. Strong social networks improve mental health and encourage healthy behaviors. Recognizing the power of community means ensuring everyone has access to supportive relationships and networks. Sometimes that involves community programs, social groups, or just opportunities to connect with others.

- **Food and Nutrition:** Food is more than just fuel—it is the foundation for energy, growth, and overall health. Access to nutritious food is essential for proper physical development, brain function, and disease prevention. Yet many people live in "food deserts" where fresh, healthy options are scarce. Example: David lives in an urban neighborhood where the nearest full grocery store is miles away, but fast-food restaurants are on every corner. Without reliable transportation, his family often relies on convenience store snacks and frozen meals high in salt and preservatives. Over time, this lack of nutritious food increases his risk of diabetes and heart disease. Food security means having consistent access to affordable, healthy meals. When people struggle to obtain nutritious food, the effects ripple into their ability to concentrate at school, their productivity at work, and their management of chronic illness. Creating equitable access to fresh produce, nutrition education, and culturally relevant food isn't just about diet—it's about laying a cornerstone of health and resilience.

- **Work and Recreation:** Work provides not only income but also shapes identity, purpose, and social connections. Recreation and leisure activities promote physical health, mental well-being, and work-life balance. Disparities in job security, workplace conditions, and access to recreational spaces can create health inequities. Example: Jessica is a hospital technician working long, irregular hours. She enjoys her work, but the stress and exhaustion leave her little energy to exercise or spend time with family. Without flexible scheduling or wellness supports, her physical and mental health suffer, leading to burnout. In contrast, Liam works at a company that prioritizes employee well-being—he has regular breaks, supportive management, and a park near the office for walks. He has time for hobbies and family, which boosts his health and productivity. Equitable policies that support a healthy work environment, along with access to parks and leisure, create conditions where people can thrive both professionally and personally.

The Interconnected Nature of SDOH: Each category of SDOH is distinct, but they are deeply interconnected, forming a web that shapes our lives. For instance, lack of economic stability can limit access to quality education, which in turn affects job opportunities and income. Living in a poorly maintained neighborhood can make it harder to access healthcare or build strong social connections. This interconnectedness means addressing one determinant often requires addressing others. It also highlights the importance of systems thinking—understanding how policies, environments, and resources interact to either support or undermine health. Throughout this toolkit, we will integrate questions and reflections that touch on multiple SDOH categories at once, because improving one area often benefits others.

As we dive deeper into SDOH, consider the "roots" of your own life. Are they firmly planted in supportive soil, or are there areas where the ground feels rocky? By examining these determinants and their impact, we can begin to nurture the soil in our lives and communities, ensuring that everyone has the opportunity to grow and thrive.

The Roots Beneath the Surface

When you look at a thriving tree, it's easy to focus on what's above ground—the branches stretching toward the sky, the leaves soaking up sunlight, the fruit it bears in season. But what we don't see, and often don't pause to consider, is the intricate network of roots beneath the surface. Those roots keep the tree alive, stable, and growing. Without healthy, deep roots, the tree cannot stand tall.

Human lives are no different. Our health and well-being are shaped by both what's visible—the choices we make or the opportunities we take—and by conditions that anchor us below the surface. These conditions—our social determinants of health—form the roots of our lives. They largely determine how we grow, adapt, and ultimately thrive.

Every person has a story shaped by the environment they're planted in. Sometimes those stories are filled with opportunity and abundance; other times, they reveal struggle and resilience in the face of barren soil.

For example, Tanya is a mother working tirelessly to keep her family afloat. Every month, as she stands in the grocery aisle making calculations, she wonders: if she spends more on fresh, nutritious food, will she fall short on rent? These decisions weigh on her, draining her energy and impacting her health. Tanya's high blood pressure didn't appear from nowhere—it's tied to the financial stress surrounding her every day.

Then there's Caleb, a teenager with a bright mind and big dreams, living in a neighborhood with few resources. His school is overcrowded, the library's books are outdated, and there are no after-school programs to nurture his interests. Across town, another student, Marcus, enjoys smaller class sizes, mentorship programs, and extracurricular activities that build confidence. Both Caleb and Marcus have potential, but the opportunities available to them are worlds apart.

These stories show how the soil we grow in—our environment, connections, and access to resources—shapes what we can imagine for ourselves. They remind us that thriving isn't only about individual effort; it's also about the support we receive from the world around us.

The Bigger Picture

When we talk about health, it's easy to focus narrowly on what happens in a doctor's office or hospital. But the truth is, the factors influencing health outcomes start long before anyone sets foot in a clinic.

- Economic stability determines whether someone can afford preventive care or fill a prescription.
- Education shapes whether they understand their diagnosis or can navigate a complex healthcare system.
- Neighborhoods and environments decide whether children have safe places to play or access to nutritious food.
- Social connection and support provide the resilience to face life's challenges.

These aren't distant, abstract concepts—they are the building blocks of our daily lives. They are often siloed in discussions of health, but in reality they merge into a single picture of well-being.

Why It Matters: A focus on SDOH isn't about assigning blame or making excuses; it's about recognizing what's happening beneath the surface. When we invest in creating environments where people like Tanya and Caleb can thrive, we aren't just improving individual lives—we're strengthening the roots of entire communities. Healthier individuals lead to healthier families, workplaces, and neighborhoods.

Addressing SDOH means shifting the question from "Why isn't this person making healthy choices?" to "What conditions would help this person (or community) flourish?" It's not about quick fixes or surface-level solutions. It's about enriching the soil so that everyone, regardless of where they start, has the chance to grow strong and healthy.

A New Perspective

Imagine what it would look like if every child had access to quality education, if every family felt financially secure, and if every neighborhood was a place where people could live and play safely. Think of what we could accomplish when everyone has the opportunity to live a full and healthy life.

This vision isn't a far-fetched dream—it's a goal worth striving for. When we focus on the roots, we don't just support individuals—we uplift whole communities. And that's what matters most.

The Start of a New Journey: The greatest secret of the human experience is this: no matter what our external environment looks like—no matter the barriers, challenges, or circumstances—we have the power to reshape it from the inside out. Change isn't always easy, but it starts with a choice, and that choice lies within each of us.

This toolkit, along with the accompanying self-assessment, is an invitation to take an intentional step. It provides tangible strategies to assess and improve the areas of your life most tied to well-being. The Social Determinants of Health are not immovable forces—they're dynamic. With the right tools, guidance, and effort, they can be reshaped to better support your life.

The Power of Internal Change: It's tempting to believe that change must begin with the world around us—that we just need better circumstances, more opportunities, or fewer barriers. But in truth, change often begins internally. It starts with the life we choose to live, the mindset we embrace, and the habits we commit to. That's the secret: by changing ourselves, we begin to change our environment.

Yet, internal change isn't a solitary act. Sometimes we need a hand to guide us, a friend to encourage us, or a tool to help us navigate unfamiliar territory. This is where the toolkit becomes invaluable. It's not just a collection of ideas; it's a roadmap to help you reflect on your current circumstances, identify areas for growth, and take actionable steps toward thriving.

Opportunities in a Connected World: We live in an era of unprecedented connection. The internet has opened doors to new communities and resources, making it possible to reshape our environments in ways previous generations could never imagine. But with this opportunity comes a challenge: the sheer volume of information can be overwhelming. Algorithms can suggest content or contacts, but they can't replace real relationships or the personal growth that comes from deliberate choices.

That's why this process can't rely solely on technology or external systems. It requires each of us to get involved in real life. Making new friends, engaging with supportive communities, seeking mentors—these are deliberate acts that create fertile ground for personal growth. This toolkit offers guidance to take those intentional steps—to bridge the gap between possibility and action.

(Join the community at tellegacy.org for more information.)

A Nudge in the Right Direction: Sometimes all it takes is a small nudge to spark a transformative journey. It might come from a friend encouraging you to take a chance, a story that resonates, or a resource (like this toolkit) that provides the tools to stay connected. The journey toward thriving in every area of your life isn't about grand, sweeping changes overnight. It's about small, deliberate choices that compound over time.

This toolkit is a nudge. It's designed to help you examine the key areas of your life that influence your health and happiness, and it offers practical suggestions for improvement. It empowers you to take control of your goals—one step at a time—in the SDOH areas that matter most to you.

The Role of Caregivers: Caregiving is one of the most profound roles a person can take on. It sits at a unique intersection of compassion, resilience, and responsibility. Whether you're caring for yourself, a loved one, or supporting others professionally (as a Community Health Worker, Social Worker, Case Manager, etc.), you stand on the front lines of transforming lives. To fulfill this role effectively, you must begin with yourself.

Start with Yourself: The Oxygen Mask Rule - You may have heard the advice on airplanes: "Put on your own oxygen mask before helping others." This isn't just emergency guidance—it's a life philosophy for caregivers. We're all caregivers in some capacity—first for ourselves, and then for others. We each have the responsibility of taking care of our own needs and also caring for others. Both sides of care are equally important. To be present and effective for those you support, you must first tend to your own well-being.

Caregiving often requires more emotional and physical energy than anticipated. It involves late nights, hard conversations, and navigating complex systems. If you neglect your own needs, burnout becomes inevitable. That's why self-care is essential—not as a luxury, but as the foundation for your ability to support others.

Taking care of yourself means finding balance. It means setting boundaries, asking for help when you need it, and prioritizing your physical and mental health. When you care for yourself, you set an example for those you support. You show them what it looks like to value well-being, which is often the first step in helping them do the same.

The Caregiver's Role in Addressing SDOH: Caregivers are often the first point of contact for someone facing challenges. You are the person others turn to when systems feel overwhelming or resources seem out of reach. This gives you profound influence as both an advocate and a connector.

- **As an advocate:** you ensure that the people in your care have a voice. Whether it's fighting for a loved one's right to quality medical care or helping someone secure affordable housing, you stand in the gap to see that their needs are met. Advocacy means seeing the potential in someone's life and working to create the conditions that allow that potential to emerge.
- **As a connector:** you link people to resources and opportunities. You might help someone navigate a confusing healthcare system, find community support, or enroll in a program they didn't know existed. This role requires patience, creativity, and a deep understanding of how systems work—and where they fall short.

Caregivers in Action: Real Stories of Impact – Caregiving doesn't look the same for everyone, but its impact is universal. Here are a few examples of caregivers addressing SDOH in meaningful ways:

- **The CHW Bridging the Gap:** In a community with limited access to fresh food, a Community Health Worker noticed families struggling to maintain healthy diets. She partnered with a local nonprofit to start a weekly produce distribution and educated families about nutrition programs. Her efforts not only provided immediate relief—they empowered families to take charge of their health.

- **The Advocate for Safe Housing:** David cared for his aging mother, who lived in an unsafe apartment with rising rent. He saw her health suffering as a result, so he researched affordable housing options and tirelessly advocated with local housing authorities. His persistence paid off when she moved into a clean, safe apartment close to her medical care.
- **The Case Manager Ensuring Follow-Up Care:** After a hospital discharge, a case manager realized her patient (who lived alone) had no transportation to follow-up appointments. She connected the patient to a ride service, ensuring their recovery wasn't derailed by missed care. This small intervention had a significant impact on the patient's long-term health.

Each of these caregivers transformed challenges into opportunities. Their actions show how addressing SDOH at an individual level can ripple outward, improving lives in lasting ways.

The Ripple Effect of Caregiving: Caregiving is a catalyst for change. The small, deliberate actions you take—helping someone access healthcare, educating them about resources, simply listening—create ripples that extend far beyond the immediate moment.

For example, if as a case manager or CHW you guide someone through enrolling in Medicaid, you reduce their financial stress and give them peace of mind, allowing them to focus on other areas of life. When you connect someone to a community group, you're not just alleviating their isolation—you're helping build a support network that strengthens their resilience.

The ripple effect of caregiving isn't just about individual lives; it uplifts entire communities. Healthier individuals contribute to stronger families, more vibrant neighborhoods, and systems that work better for everyone.

Equipping Yourself for the Journey: Whether you are caring for yourself, a child, an aging parent, or clients in a professional capacity, remember that you have a remarkable ability to create change. To sustain this work, however, you need tools, knowledge, and support. That's where this SDOH toolkit comes in. It's designed to help you:

- Reflect on the key areas of SDOH and how they affect those you care for.
- Develop practical strategies to address barriers and create opportunities.
- Strengthen your own resilience so you can continue to show up with purpose and compassion.

Perhaps you picked up this toolkit because you know caregiving is not a role you need to navigate alone. With the right support, we can amplify our impact and create lasting change for the people and communities we serve.

Your Legacy of Care: The work of caregivers often goes unnoticed, but its impact is profound. Every act of compassion, advocacy, and connection leaves a legacy that shapes lives for generations. By helping individuals overcome challenges and nurturing their potential to thrive, you are nourishing the roots of our shared human garden.

The strength of a tree comes from its roots, and as caregivers, we nourish those roots. Our work creates the conditions for growth, resilience, and transformation. That role is of extraordinary significance.

Reflection and Action: Staying Connected to the Soil

Let's pause here. You've spent time exploring the foundations of SDOH and how they shape lives—yours included. We've seen that each of us is part of a bigger ecosystem, rooted in connections and environments that sustain us. (As an aside, even the author writing this is a natural introvert who has learned the value of staying connected.)

Think of yourself as that plant we spoke about earlier. You aren't meant to thrive in isolation, and you shouldn't expect to. Your strength, growth, and ability to weather life's storms come from being connected to the soil of your relationships and community. Take a moment to reflect on how those connections shape your everyday life and what it might mean to care for them intentionally.

Consider:

- **Who are the people in your life who act as the "soil" for your well-being?** Think about the relationships that give you strength and nourishment.
- **Are there areas in your life where the soil feels dry or depleted?** What could it look like to "water" those areas—to reach out, reconnect, or deepen a relationship?

- **What does staying rooted mean to you personally?** What practices or habits help you feel connected, supported, and steady?

This reflection isn't about "fixing" anything right now or rushing to act. It's about letting these ideas sink in. Internally acknowledge the value of your relationships, your community, and your role within them. You and I are part of something bigger, and that connection—like the roots of a tree in healthy soil—has the potential to help us thrive in ways we might not yet see.

Remember, we're walking this path together. Each step of the journey is an opportunity to uncover what nourishes you, what strengthens your roots, and how you can stay connected to the soil that sustains your life. Take your time. The answers will come as you reflect, observe, and grow.

Call to Action: Understanding SDOH as a Foundation for Change - We've laid the groundwork. Together, we've uncovered how SDOH influence the environments we live in, the choices available to us, and the relationships that give our lives texture and meaning. This knowledge is powerful. It marks the starting point of a movement toward intentional change—change that reaches beyond individual well-being and touches the systems and communities we're part of. When we understand the roots of health, we begin to shift what's possible—for ourselves and for those we care about.

Think back to the image of the plant and the soil. Now picture yourself as someone who not only tends to your own roots but also helps enrich the soil around you. You may be a caregiver, a community advocate, or simply someone trying to create better conditions for your loved ones. Whatever your role, your understanding of SDOH equips you to make a difference.

Your Role in the Bigger Picture: Change doesn't usually start with grand gestures. Often, it begins with small, intentional steps—observing, reflecting, and deciding how to act. As you move forward, you might realize that the power to create pathways for resilience and equity is already in your hands, right now.

When you help someone feel seen, when you advocate for a resource that might otherwise go unnoticed, or when you connect someone to opportunities they didn't know existed, you are cultivating the foundation for growth and transformation. Each action adds richness to the soil, creating space for others—and yourself—to thrive.

Let's Continue Together: The work you do matters. It matters on the hard days, the busy days, and the days when the impact isn't immediately visible. By deepening your understanding of SDOH, you are opening doors—for yourself, for those you serve, and for your wider community.

Resilience is built in small, quiet moments. Equity grows when we choose to see gaps and step forward to address them. Better outcomes come from intentionality, persistence, and connection. This makes your role vital.

Let's keep walking this path together, step by step, with purpose and care. This is just the beginning of the journey, but it's one worth taking—because the seeds we plant today will shape a future where everyone has the chance to thrive. (In the next section, we will take the SDOH self-assessment to see where we currently stand on the SDOH scale.)

SECTION 2

SDOH SELF-ASSESSMENT (THE SDOH TEST)

Setting the Stage: The Power of Reflection

Imagine sitting with someone who truly cares about you—not asking questions to judge or analyze, but to genuinely understand. With curiosity and warmth, they lean in and ask: "How are you doing, really? What feels steady in your life, and what feels uncertain?" That is the spirit of this self-assessment.

Measurement and evaluation are important, but the main goal here is to create a habit of reflection. This survey is an invitation to step back, take stock, and ask yourself: **How are the foundations of my life affecting my health, opportunities, and potential?**

The Social Determinants of Health survey (available on our website at Tellegacy.org) is built to help you explore these very questions. Think of it as a mirror, allowing you to see where you feel strong and supported and where there might be room for growth. This clarity is the first step in creating meaningful change—whether for yourself, your loved ones, or the people you serve.

Clarity is the first step.

A Snapshot of SDOH

SDOH represent the conditions that influence our lives beyond what happens in a doctor's office. They are the building blocks of health and well-being, and they fall into seven key categories:

- **Economic Stability:** Your financial foundation—whether your resources meet your needs and give you a sense of security.
- **Education Access and Quality:** The doors opened by learning—how education shapes opportunities, health literacy, and empowerment.
- **Healthcare Access and Quality:** The ease and quality of accessing care when needed—not just having insurance, but also having culturally competent care close to home.
- **Neighborhood and Built Environment:** Your surroundings—housing quality, green spaces, safety, and access to necessities like groceries and transportation.
- **Social and Community Context:** The relationships and connections that sustain you. Who is part of your "soil," nourishing and supporting your growth?
- **Food and Nutrition:** Your access to nutritious, affordable, and culturally relevant food. Does your environment support a diet that fuels health and longevity?

- **Work and Recreation:** How your work and leisure time shape your physical and mental well-being. Does your job provide stability and purpose? Do you have outlets to recharge and find joy?

Each of these categories is intertwined. A challenge in one area often ripples into others, creating barriers to health and equity. For example, limited access to grocery stores can lead to poor nutrition, raising the risk of chronic conditions like diabetes. This doesn't just affect individuals—it widens health disparities across communities.

Organizations like Healthy People 2030 emphasize the importance of addressing these upstream factors, urging us to create social, physical, and economic environments that enable people to reach their full potential. The SDOH survey aligns with that mission, offering a way to explore how these factors appear in your life.

The Survey as an Opportunity for Insight

Completing this survey is more than checking boxes or answering questions. It's a moment to pause and consider the foundations of your life. Think of it as sitting down with yourself and asking meaningful questions about the roots of your health and well-being.

This process isn't about being perfect or having everything figured out. It's about seeing clearly—identifying where you feel steady and where you'd like to grow. The survey invites you to reflect on questions like:

- Do I feel financially secure, or am I often worried about making ends meet?

- How does my neighborhood shape my health? Does it feel like a place where I can thrive?
- Who are the people in my life who support me, and how can I nurture those connections?

There's no need to rush through this. Find a quiet space where you can reflect honestly without distractions. This isn't about anyone else—it's about you, your story, and your journey.

Reflection: Deepening Your Insights

As you complete the survey, you might feel a range of emotions—gratitude for areas of your life that feel stable, or frustration for areas that feel less secure. All these feelings are valid and part of the process.

Remember, this is just your starting point. Like tending a garden, the goal isn't to have everything perfect immediately. It's to understand where the soil needs enriching, where the roots need watering, and where new growth is possible.

SDOH: A Foundation for Change

By the end of this survey, you'll have a clearer picture of how SDOH manifest in your life. You'll see which areas feel like fertile ground and which might need a little more care.

The survey helps identify areas where you can begin to make changes, however small. It also prepares you to better understand and support others, whether that's your family, your clients, or your community. You'll find that the work you do to improve these areas in your life can ripple outward, creating paths to resilience and equity for those around you.

Why Emotional Safety Matters

Emotional safety is the foundation for honest reflection and meaningful change. When we feel safe discussing vulnerable aspects of our lives—like finances, housing, or access to healthcare—we create space to acknowledge what's working and what isn't, without fear of judgment. That kind of openness is powerful. It shifts the focus from blame or shame to understanding and possibility. This survey is designed with that principle in mind. It's not about fixing everything at once or achieving perfection. It's about cultivating awareness and connection—within yourself and with those you support.

When we take time to explore our emotional landscape, we open doors to transformation. And when we create that same safety for others—whether a loved one, a client, or a community member—we give them the conditions they need to thrive. Emotional safety isn't just a nice concept; it's an essential element of growth, resilience, and lasting change.

An Invitation to Grow

The Social Determinants of Health are complex, interconnected, and deeply personal. They affect nearly everyone in some way, shaping our health, our opportunities, and our experiences. By taking this survey, you're taking a step toward awareness and change.

What matters is what we decide to do each day with that knowledge. Every reflection, every question answered, is a seed planted. Over time, as you nurture those seeds, you'll find that growth and transformation are possible.

Take your time with this process. Approach it with curiosity, warmth, and a sense of purpose. Completing this survey means you're stepping into a journey of growth, resilience, and possibility. Let's take that step together.

The Seven Categories of the SDOH Test and Their Questions

The seven Social Determinants of Health represent vital parts of life's foundation. Together, they provide a framework for understanding how our environments, relationships, and resources shape health, opportunity, and well-being. The survey invites you to reflect on each category through supportive questions, encouraging you to explore both strengths and areas for growth.

The survey uses a 7-point response scale, ranging from "To a Very Great Extent" to "Not at All." This range lets you gauge how much each area contributes to your well-being (or creates stress), and it provides clear benchmarks for self-awareness and action.

The survey is designed to clearly show how one area can affect another. You may notice that a question about financial stability also appears in the healthcare section, or a question about your neighborhood appears in the economic stability section. This is intentional—it reflects how each part of our life influences the others. When you complete the survey, you'll receive a score for each category along with recommendations on how you can strengthen those areas over time.

(We recommend taking the SDOH Test once a week for the next 8–10 weeks as you gradually work on goals to improve your scores.) Remember, you're not alone on this journey. Our team is here to help you set goals and achieve them one by one. We're here to assist you in pursuing progress without the burden of figuring everything out by yourself. You can always

contact us at **social@tellegacy.com** or via the "**Contact Us**" page at **tellegacy.org**. You are not alone.

How to Take the Survey & What Happens Next

Accessing the Survey: You can complete the full SDOH survey on our website. Visit tellegacy.org and look for the SDOH Test. Keep in mind, this isn't about getting a "good" or "bad" score—it's about understanding your strengths and finding opportunities to grow.

Once you complete the survey, you'll receive immediate results: your scores in each category and practical steps you can take to improve in each area. Whether you're looking for small tweaks or big changes, these tailored recommendations will help you move forward confidently.

And if you ever want extra support, our team is here. Whether you need guidance, additional resources, or one-on-one help, you'll have access to professionals ready to assist you in raising your scores as high as you'd like.

This is not about pressure. It's about possibility. Wherever you are right now, there's always room to grow, and always a way forward. We're on this journey with you.

Taking the SDOH Test on Tellegacy.org – A Quick Guide

Step 1: Access the SDOH Test – Open your browser and go to tellegacy.org. Navigate the menu or homepage to find the Social Determinants of Health Test, and click on it to begin.

Step 2: Provide Basic Information – Before starting the assessment, you'll be asked for some basic demographic details to personalize your results. This may include:

- Name
- Email address (to receive results or follow-up resources)
- Age, gender, and race
- Education level and profession
- City, state, and country

These details help contextualize your responses and may allow for tailored insights, but remember that your survey responses remain confidential.

Step 3: Answer the SDOH Questions – The test consists of questions across different life domains. Each question uses a Likert scale where you rate your response from "To a Very Great Extent" to "Not at All."

Categories and Sample Questions:

- **Economic Stability** – e.g., "Can you afford nutritious food consistently?"
- **Education Access & Quality** – e.g., "Do you have resources to support learning and career growth?"
- **Healthcare Access & Quality** – e.g., "Can you receive medical care without significant financial stress?"
- **Neighborhood & Built Environment** – e.g., "Does your community offer safe spaces and essential services?"

- **Social & Community Context** – e.g., "Do you feel a sense of belonging and emotional support?"
- **Food & Nutrition** – e.g., "Are affordable, healthy food options available in your area?"
- **Work & Recreation** – e.g., "Does your job or volunteering provide fulfillment, and do you have opportunities to recharge?"

Select the response that best represents your experience for each question.

Step 4: Submit the Test – Review your answers for accuracy, then click the submit button at the end of the assessment. Wait for confirmation—depending on the system, you may see instant feedback on screen and/or receive an email with insights.

Step 5: Interpret & Use Your Results:- Identify strengths and gaps in your social determinants of health.- Use your insights to seek out resources that improve your well-being.- Consider sharing your results with healthcare providers, social workers, or community support groups to get further assistance.

Completing the SDOH Test on Tellegacy.org is a quick and effective way to evaluate how key life factors influence your overall well-being. By taking a few minutes to answer thoughtfully, you gain a comprehensive perspective on your health and social environment.

What You'll See After Clicking "Submit"

Once you complete the SDOH Test and click "Submit," the results page will give you a detailed breakdown of your responses. This summary helps you understand how different aspects of your environment and lifestyle contribute to your overall well-being. Here's what to expect:

- **Overview of Results:** At the top, you'll see a summary of the personal information you entered (like name, profession, location, etc.) for reference. These details do not affect your score or recommendations; they're just for context.
- **Total SDOH Score:** You'll see a total cumulative score (out of a maximum of 392 points, since each of the 7 categories has a maximum score of 56). This number is the sum of all your category scores, giving you an overall snapshot. (A perfect score indicates the highest level of satisfaction and access across all categories. A lower score suggests areas where improvement may be needed.)
- **Breakdown of Scores by Category:** Your results will be divided into the seven categories of SDOH, each showing:
- Your score in that category (e.g., **Economic Stability: 33/56**).
- A benchmark rating categorizing your satisfaction level, such as "Very Satisfied," "Satisfied," "Moderately Satisfied," etc. For example:
- (This is an example. Each benchmark gives a sense of how well your current environment supports your well-being in that category.)

Interpretation of Your Scores:

- Higher scores (closer to 56 per category) suggest you have strong support and access to resources in that area.

- Moderate scores indicate some aspects are working well, but there may be challenges to address.
- Lower scores (closer to 0) suggest a lack of access, opportunities, or satisfaction in that area.

A refined satisfaction scale for reference might look like this:- 51–56: Extremely Satisfied- 45–50: Very Satisfied- 39–44: Satisfied- 33–38: Moderately Satisfied- 27–32: Somewhat Satisfied- 21–26: Slightly Satisfied- 15–20: Neutral- 9–14: Dissatisfied- 3–8: Very Dissatisfied- 1–2: Extremely Dissatisfied

- **Recommendations for Improvement:** Based on your score in each category, you will receive general guidance on how to improve your well-being in areas where your score is lower. While exact recommendations depend on your answers, they may include suggestions like:
- *Economic Stability:* Tips for accessing financial planning resources, job training programs, or community support services.
- *Education Access & Quality:* Information on scholarships, mentorship opportunities, or educational resources in your area.
- *Healthcare Access & Quality:* Strategies to navigate healthcare services, find affordable care options, or advocate for better support.
- *Neighborhood & Environment:* Advice on community engagement, housing options, or local advocacy to improve safety and resources.

- *Social & Community Context:* Encouragement to strengthen personal relationships, seek out support groups, or engage in community-building activities.
- *Food & Nutrition:* Ideas for accessing nutritious food, meal planning on a budget, or finding local food assistance programs.
- *Work & Recreation:* Ideas for enhancing work-life balance, finding fulfilling activities outside of work, or improving job satisfaction.
- **Version Information:** At the bottom of the results page, you might see a note like "Release 1.0," indicating the version of the survey system.

The purpose of these questions and results is to create a safe space to pause, reflect, and understand your life in greater depth. Now, let's dive deeper into the survey questions by category, beginning with Economic Stability.

Economic Stability

Economic stability forms the bedrock of many aspects of life. It's about more than income, it speaks to the peace of mind that comes from knowing your basic needs are covered and your future is within reach. When this financial foundation feels steady, it's easier to engage fully in other areas of life, like housing, healthcare, nutrition, and relationships. You can plan, rest, and face life's challenges with greater confidence, knowing you have support to navigate what comes your way.

Reflect on the following questions about your economic stability, keeping emotional safety in mind. This is a space to explore your relationship with financial security without judgment—just curiosity and care:

- Do you have access to educational resources or training opportunities that help you achieve your financial goals? (Education Access and Quality)
- Does your financial situation enable you to access quality healthcare services without significant stress? (Healthcare Access and Quality)
- Does your neighborhood provide opportunities or resources that help you achieve financial stability? (Neighborhood and Built Environment)
- Do you have someone you trust to discuss your financial goals and challenges—someone who provides emotional or practical support? (Social and Community Context)
- Can you consistently afford healthy and nutritious food for yourself and your family? (Food and Nutrition)
- Does your current economic situation allow you to engage in meaningful work or recreational activities that bring you fulfillment? (Work and Recreation)
- **Overall Stress Level:** How would you rate your stress level related to your financial situation? What is the primary source of that stress, if any?

Why This Matters: Economic stability is more than numbers on a paycheck—it's about the freedom to focus on what matters most, from personal growth to supporting loved ones. When financial concerns are overwhelming, they can overshadow other parts of life, creating barriers to health, happy moments, and connection. Reflecting on this category helps you see how your financial situation supports, or limits, your well-being. Whether you're thriving, struggling, or somewhere in between, this process is an opportunity to recognize where you are now and imagine what growth could look like.

Take your time with these questions, and remember: this isn't about fixing everything at once. It's about building awareness, one thoughtful step at a time. With that awareness, you'll have the tools to nurture meaningful change in your life and the lives of others.

Your Next Steps (Economic Stability): Once you've reflected on these questions (and those that follow in later categories), think about what stands out. Were there areas where you feel strong and supported? Were there places where you wish you had more access, encouragement, or resources?

Education Access and Quality: Expanding Your Opportunities

When we think about education, we often think of degrees, diplomas, or formal training. But education is really about access, access to knowledge, new perspectives, and skills that shape how we navigate life. It's about feeling equipped to make informed decisions, pursue meaningful work, and take on new challenges with confidence.

No matter where you are in your journey, education remains a powerful tool for growth. It can open doors, shift mindsets, and provide the foundation for greater opportunities. We're not here to measure whether you've done "enough" in the past. We're here, together, to explore how education has shaped our lives and where we might want to expand our understanding going forward. It's about discovering where we might want to continue learning, in whatever way makes sense for us.

Take your time with these questions, and be honest about what feels strong and what might need more support:

Reflect on how education has played a role in your life—whether through formal schooling, professional training, mentorship, or even personal experiences that taught you valuable lessons.

- Does your financial situation impact your ability to pursue educational opportunities or training? (Economic Stability)
- Has your education prepared you to make informed decisions about your health and access healthcare effectively? (Healthcare Access and Quality)
- Do local resources (like libraries, internet access, or community programs) support your educational goals? (Neighborhood and Built Environment)
- Do you have a support system (family, friends, or mentors) that encourages and motivates you to pursue education or training? (Social and Community Context)
- Does your access to education include programs or resources on maintaining good nutrition and health? (Food and Nutrition)
- Has your education prepared you for meaningful work or fulfilling recreational activities that align with your goals? (Work and Recreation)
- Overall Stress Level: How stressful is your current educational situation or lack of access? What contributes most to your stress in this area, if anything?

(Think about formal or informal education: it could be school, workshops, online courses, or learning from others.)

Healthcare Access and Quality: The Gateway to Well-Being

What do you think of when you consider "healthcare"? Day to day, we might reduce healthcare to an appointment on a calendar or a medication refill. But let's think of it in broader terms: healthcare as feeling supported, informed, and confident in your ability to care for yourself. Access to quality healthcare brings peace of mind, ensuring help is within reach when you need guidance, treatment, or preventive care.

Think about the last time you had a question about your health. Did you feel you had someone to turn to? Were you able to find the answers and care you needed? Research shows that when people feel empowered in their healthcare decisions, they make choices that support long-term well-being. Feeling informed about your options, having a provider you trust, and knowing that healthcare fits within your life and budget all contribute to a sense of security and vitality.

This section will help you reflect on what's working well in your healthcare access and where you might want to explore new possibilities for even better support:

As you consider these questions, reflect on how you feel about your access to care, the quality of information available to you, and whether your healthcare experience supports the life you want to live:

- Do you have the financial means (such as insurance or other support) to access necessary healthcare services without significant hardship? (Economic Stability)

- Do you feel informed and educated about accessing healthcare services and making decisions about your health? (Education Access and Quality)
- Are there quality healthcare providers or facilities easily accessible in your neighborhood or community? (Neighborhood and Built Environment)
- Do you have someone you trust to help you navigate healthcare decisions or provide support during health-related challenges? (Social and Community Context)
- Do you have access to nutritional support or counseling to help maintain or improve your health? (Food and Nutrition)
- Does your healthcare access support your ability to work or participate in recreational activities without undue stress or limitations? (Work and Recreation)
- **Overall Stress Level:** How stressful do you find managing your healthcare needs, if at all?

Neighborhood and Built Environment: The Spaces That Support Us

This section invites you to step back and look at how your neighborhood contributes to your well-being. What's working? What could be better?

As you consider the questions below, reflect on how your neighborhood supports your financial, social, and personal well-being. Think about what aspects you appreciate most and where you might want new opportunities:

- Does your neighborhood offer opportunities for financial growth or stability, such as jobs or affordable living options? (Economic Stability)

- Are there resources in your neighborhood that support education or skill development, such as schools, libraries, or reliable internet access? (Education Access and Quality)
- Is there adequate access to quality healthcare services, pharmacies, or wellness programs in your neighborhood? (Healthcare Access and Quality)
- Do you feel a sense of community and safety in your neighborhood that supports your overall well-being? (Social and Community Context)
- Can you access affordable and nutritious food options within your neighborhood? (Food and Nutrition)
- Does your neighborhood provide opportunities for meaningful work or recreational activities that support your personal or professional goals? (Work and Recreation)
- **Overall Stress Level:** How stressful do you find living in your neighborhood, if at all?

Social and Community Context: The Power of Connection

The people around us—friends, family, mentors, coworkers, neighbors—shape our experiences in ways we might take for granted. Think about a time when someone's kindness lifted your spirits, when a conversation gave you a new perspective, or when a friend's encouragement gave you the confidence to take a leap. That's the power of connection.

Connection isn't just about being surrounded by people, it's about feeling truly supported. Do you have people in your life who encourage your dreams? Who stand by you when life gets tough? Who make you feel seen and valued?

This section invites you to reflect on the relationships in your life—where they bring joy and where you might want to deepen your connections:

As you consider these questions, focus on the role your relationships play in your everyday life. Consider not only who supports you, but also how you feel within your communities:

- Do you have people in your life who provide emotional or practical support for achieving financial stability or economic goals? (Economic Stability)
- Does your social network encourage your educational growth or provide resources for lifelong learning? (Education Access and Quality)
- Are there individuals in your social circle who help you navigate healthcare decisions or support you during health challenges? (Healthcare Access and Quality)
- Do you feel a sense of belonging and connection in your community or neighborhood? (Neighborhood and Built Environment)
- Do you have people who support you in maintaining a healthy diet or who can help you access nutritious food when needed? (Food and Nutrition)
- Do you feel supported by your social or professional network in pursuing meaningful work or recreational activities? (Work and Recreation)
- **Overall Stress Level:** How stressful do you find maintaining your social relationships, if at all?

Your Next Steps (Social Connections): Strong relationships don't happen by accident—they're built with intention, care, and time. If your support system feels strong, celebrate that and continue nurturing those connections. If you're looking for more support, know there are always ways to expand and deepen your community. Remember, when you complete the survey online, you'll receive insights into how your social and community context shapes your life—along with practical ways to strengthen your connections and build a support system that uplifts you.

Food and Nutrition: Fueling Your Body, Nourishing Your Life

Hungry? We all love a good meal. But food is more than just fuel—it's also connection, comfort, culture, and a foundation for our health and energy. Think about the best meal you've ever had. Maybe it was a home-cooked dish made with love, a vibrant meal shared with friends, or something simple that just made you feel good. Food has the power to nourish us not only physically, but emotionally and socially as well.

What we eat affects everything: our mood, energy, focus, and long-term health. Research from the Harvard T.H. Chan School of Public Health shows that a diet rich in whole foods, fruits, and vegetables reduces the risk of chronic diseases and improves mental clarity and emotional well-being. Consistent access to nutritious foods makes our bodies and minds better equipped to take on the day, pursue our goals, and fully engage in life.

Maintaining a healthy diet isn't only about knowing what's good for you. It's also about having access to the right foods, feeling supported in your choices, and ensuring that food brings nourishment rather than stress. This section invites you to reflect on how food and nutrition fit into your life right now and where you might create more ease and balance:

As you think through these questions, consider how your food choices and eating habits impact your daily life—physically, emotionally, and socially:

- Do you have the financial means to consistently purchase nutritious and sufficient food for yourself and your family? (Economic Stability)
- Do you have adequate knowledge or education about maintaining a healthy diet and its benefits? (Education Access and Quality)
- Do you have access to nutritional counseling or programs that support your health needs? (Healthcare Access and Quality)
- Are there affordable and nutritious food options in your neighborhood or community? (Neighborhood and Built Environment)
- Do you have a support system that helps you maintain healthy eating habits or provides food when you're in need? (Social and Community Context)
- Does your access to food support your energy and well-being so you can engage in work or recreational activities without feeling fatigued or unhealthy? (Work and Recreation)
- **Overall Stress Level:** How stressful is it for you to obtain or maintain access to nutritious food? What is the primary source of stress, if any?

Your Next Steps (Food & Nutrition): Food is one of the most essential aspects of well-being, and everyone deserves access to nourishing, satisfying meals that support a vibrant life. If you feel strong in this area, take a moment to appreciate that—you're giving yourself and your body what it needs to thrive. If there are areas where you'd like more stability or knowledge, know that there are resources and strategies to help make healthy eating easier and more accessible.

Work and Recreation: Purpose, Passion, and Play

Work and recreation shape the rhythm of our days and influence our sense of purpose, fulfillment, and overall well-being. Think about the career you've built, the hobbies that bring you joy, or any spiritual or leisure practices that ground you. These activities form a core part of who we are.

Work provides more than a paycheck—it can be a source of growth, stability, and contribution. At the same time, recreation, rest, and creative outlets are crucial for maintaining balance and resilience. According to research from the Global Wellness Institute, people who feel a sense of purpose in their work and engage in fulfilling recreational activities report lower stress, higher energy, and greater life satisfaction. The key isn't just working or just relaxing, it's about alignment. Do the ways you spend your time nourish you?

Holistic health experts and organizations like the National Center for Complementary and Integrative Health suggest that integrating mindful practices, through fulfilling work, creative hobbies, physical movement, or spiritual engagement—leads to improved emotional and physical health. Whether it's journaling, gardening, meditation, or simply taking a walk in nature, these small choices contribute to a life that feels both grounded and expansive.

This section invites you to reflect on how work and recreation fit into your life. Do they energize you? Do they align with what matters most to you? By understanding where you feel fulfilled and where you might want more balance, you can take steps toward creating a life that is both meaningful and sustainable.

As you consider these questions, think about your work, the activities you enjoy, and how you spend your time. Consider whether these areas align with your values, goals, and well-being:

- Does your work provide financial stability and allow you to meet your economic goals? (If you're retired, consider whether your retirement income provides financial stability.) (Economic Stability)
- Has your education adequately prepared you for your current work or recreational pursuits? (Education Access and Quality)
- Do your physical and mental health allow you to fully engage in meaningful work, activities, or recreation? (Healthcare Access and Quality)
- Are there opportunities in your community for recreational or work-related activities that bring you fulfillment? (Neighborhood and Built Environment)
- Do you feel supported by coworkers, mentors, or friends in your work or recreational activities? (Social and Community Context)
- Do you feel your access to nutritious food supports your energy and well-being for work and recreation? (Food and Nutrition)

- **Overall Stress Level:** How stressful is it for you to manage your work and recreational activities? What contributes most to that stress, if any?

Your Next Steps (Work & Recreation): Life is richer when our work aligns with our values and when we make time for activities that bring us joy. Whether you love what you do, are working toward something new, or are seeking better balance, use this reflection to check in with yourself.

When you complete the full survey online, you'll gain insights into how your work and recreation contribute to your overall well-being, along with practical steps to create more fulfillment, energy, and joy in this area of your life. If you want to explore career development, creative outlets, or ways to bring more meaning into your daily activities, remember that resources and support are available to help.

Your work and recreation should add to your life, not deplete it. You have the right to wake up feeling excited about what you're creating, whether through your job, your passions, or the moments that restore you. Let this be an invitation to build a life where purpose and play go hand in hand.

Bringing It All Together: How SDOH Shape a Balanced Life

After completing the survey, you will see more clearly how economic stability, education, healthcare, neighborhood, social connections, food, and work/recreation are not separate, isolated aspects of life. They are deeply interconnected, shaping our well-being, opportunities, and experiences.

Think about a thriving garden. It's not just about the soil, or the water, or the sunlight, it's about how all these elements interact to support growth. When the conditions are right, plants flourish. When something is missing, nutrients in the soil, access to water, enough space to grow, the garden struggles. The same is true in our lives. When one area is thriving, it strengthens the others. When one area is struggling, it can influence everything else.

Let's examine how these elements work together through real-life examples, research, and an invitation to reflect on the balance in your own life.

Practical Next Steps After Reviewing Your SDOH Survey Results

After looking at your SDOH survey results, the next step is to take meaningful action: strengthen areas where your score was lower, while maintaining and enhancing areas where you are thriving. Below is a structured action plan to help you make progress based on your results.

- **Reflect on Your Scores:** Look at which categories scored the highest and which were moderate or lower. Ask yourself:
- Which areas feel most urgent to improve?
- Which areas do I feel I have some control over or can change right now?

The next chapter will help you explore your results, set goals, and take actionable steps toward your desired life. But before moving on—take this moment for yourself. You've started something important by reflecting on your life through this survey. Change often begins with simply noticing what needs attention.

Let's begin.

SECTION 3

REFLECTING ON SCORES AND STRENGTHENING PERSONAL SDOH

If you're here, then you've completed at least one SDOH Test. Now, let's explore some principles that will help us improve and maintain these scores. Think of this as an ongoing journey, one of delightful continuous improvement that can continue throughout our lives.

Growth Is a Journey, Not a Destination

Psychologist Dr. Carol Dweck spent decades studying what makes people thrive. Through her research on growth mindset, she discovered something simple yet profound: our potential is not fixed, it expands when we embrace life as a series of learning experiences rather than a series of pass-or-fail moments.

Dr. Dweck found that people who believe they can grow through effort and reflection tend to approach challenges with curiosity rather than fear. They see setbacks as temporary, skills as learnable, and goals as achievable through effort rather than predetermined by talent or luck. Her research shows that when we treat every experience, good or bad, as an opportunity to learn, we become more resilient, more open to possibilities, and ultimately more fulfilled.

This mindset isn't just for students in a classroom or professionals climbing a career ladder; it's for all of us, in every part of life. It applies to well-being too. When we adopt a growth mindset about our well-being, we understand that our circumstances today don't define what's possible tomorrow.

That's what this moment is about. Your survey results are not a final grade, they reflect where you are right now in this season of life. Some areas may feel strong, and others may need more attention. The beautiful thing about self-reflection is that it allows us to step into growth with awareness and intention.

Step One: Noticing What Feels Strong

Before we look at what could change, take a moment to honor what's already working well for you.

Each of us has areas in life where we feel stable, confident, or well-supported. Recognizing these strengths helps us understand what's working and how we can build on it step by step, day by day. For example:

- If your Economic Stability score reflects financial security, you likely have more options and flexibility in shaping other areas of your life, such as your health and education.
- If your Social and Community Context score demonstrates strong connections, you likely have people in your life who encourage and support you, which can help you grow in personal and professional areas.

- If your Work and Recreation score indicates fulfillment, it means the way you spend your time aligns with your sense of joy and purpose.

In positive psychology, researchers emphasize focusing on strengths rather than only trying to "fix" weaknesses. Studies from the University of Pennsylvania's Positive Psychology Center show that people who regularly acknowledge their strengths tend to be more motivated, confident, and successful in reaching their goals.

So, pause and ask yourself: **What areas of my life feel most aligned and fulfilling? How can I use these strengths to support growth in other areas?** (Write down or mentally note your reflections.)

Step Two: Identifying Areas for Growth, Without Judgment

Everyone—no matter how successful, educated, or accomplished—has areas they want to strengthen. Recognizing these areas isn't a sign of weakness; it's an invitation to grow.

Instead of seeing certain scores as "low," consider them signals pointing to where change is possible. The clearer we see where support, change, or new habits are needed, the more empowered we are to act.

Research from the National Wellness Institute shows that when people reframe challenges as opportunities for growth, they are significantly more likely to take action and create lasting change. For instance, if your Healthcare Access score is on the lower side, think about small steps to connect with better resources or begin advocating for your needs. If your Neighborhood and Built Environment score is low (perhaps reflecting limited opportunities in your area), maybe you could explore new community resources or groups. If your Food and Nutrition score suggests you struggle with maintaining a healthy diet, start looking for tools or systems that support healthier food choices.

One of the most powerful things we can do is shift our perspective from feeling stuck to seeing a path forward. That shift starts with acknowledging that every challenge carries an opportunity for growth.

Reflection question: **Which area of my life would benefit most from small, intentional improvements? What might those improvements look like?**

Step Three: Setting Small, Meaningful Goals

Research on habit formation by Dr. BJ Fogg at Stanford University finds that people are much more likely to sustain long-term change when they start small. Big, sweeping transformations can feel exciting at first, but they often become overwhelming and hard to maintain. The real key to lasting change is small, consistent actions.

If you want to build social connections, you could start by contacting a friend or neighbor to catch up. If your work-life balance feels off, set aside one hour a week for something that restores you. If you aim to eat healthier, start by adding one extra serving of vegetables a day, or replacing one sugary drink with water.

The beauty of starting small is that one positive action leads to another. Over time, these small steps create momentum—and before you know it, you've made significant progress in a natural, sustainable way.

Reflection question: **What is one simple action I can take this week to improve an area of my well-being?** (It could be as simple as going to bed 30 minutes earlier, taking a short walk at lunchtime, or calling a friend instead of scrolling on social media.)

Step Four: Recognizing the Power of Interconnection

Each area of well-being—economic stability, education, healthcare, neighborhood, social connections, food, and work/recreation, doesn't exist in isolation. They function like a thriving ecosystem: when one area grows stronger, others naturally benefit.

This means that if you improve your economic stability, you might also gain more healthcare choices, food options, and personal development opportunities. If you invest in your social and community connections, you build a support network that makes other challenges easier to manage. If you prioritize recreation and rest, you'll be better able to show up fully in other aspects of your life (like work or caregiving).

Instead of seeing these areas as separate categories, start thinking about how they work together to create balance and well-being in your life.

Consider:

- When you improve your **Economic Stability**, you create more choices for healthcare, food, and personal development.
- When you invest in **Social and Community Connections**, you gain a network of support that makes other challenges more manageable.

- When you prioritize **Recreation and Rest**, you increase your capacity to show up fully in other aspects of life.

Reflection question: **How does strengthening one area of my life create positive change in others?** (For instance, if you got a better job, how might that affect your stress levels, health habits, or relationships? If you made a new friend or joined a group, how might that affect your mental health or motivation in other areas?)

Your Strengths, Your Growth, Your Journey

The fact that you are here, reflecting and considering next steps, means you are already growing. That's something to celebrate.

Every person's journey looks different. There is no "perfect balance," only the balance that works for you. If you ever feel overwhelmed, come back to three simple questions:

1. What am I already doing well?
2. Where do I want to grow?
3. What is one small step I can take today that aligns with the life I want to create?

This is not about pressure—it's about possibility. Growth is always available to you, and every moment of awareness brings you closer to the life you want.

Final reflection question for this section: **How can I approach my personal growth with curiosity, compassion, and confidence?**

(There's no rush in answering these. They're here to guide your mindset as you proceed.)

The roadmap is yours. And the best part? The next step is entirely yours to take.

Now, let's delve into each SDOH category and discuss how to strengthen them with practical strategies and real-world examples.

Economic Stability: Building a Practical Foundation for Possibility

Financial well-being often involves earning a paycheck, but it's really about creating options, choices, and a sense of control over the practical aspects of your future. It means knowing that when a financial challenge comes—and they always do—you have the stability to navigate it. It also means that when opportunities arise, you have the flexibility to seize them.

Research by Dr. Michael Norton on the psychology of money reveals that it's not just how much money people have that impacts their well-being—it's whether they feel in control of it. His studies found that when people understand their financial situation and take intentional steps to manage it, they experience greater happiness, even at lower income levels.

In other words, the path to financial confidence doesn't require an overnight transformation. It starts with small, intentional steps that add up over time.

The Potential of Economic Stability in Everyday Life:

Let's consider Sarah's story (an example introduced earlier). Sarah is a single mother working full-time while trying to build a better future for herself and her son. She dreams of returning to school to increase her earning potential, but her paycheck barely covers rent, food, and childcare each month.

She often feels stuck—like no matter how hard she works, she's always one step behind.

Then one day, Sarah meets with a career coach at a local workforce center. The coach tells her about an online certification program that aligns with her interests and takes only six months to complete. Sarah's first reaction is skepticism—how could she afford it? But with guidance, she learns about tuition assistance programs and finds a part-time weekend job opportunity that gives her time to study in the evenings.

She starts small: one class at a time, one financial step at a time. Slowly, she sees a shift. Six months later, she earns her certification and applies for a new job. The pay increase isn't huge, but it's enough. Enough to build a small savings cushion. Enough to breathe a little easier. Enough to show her that her future isn't determined by where she started, but by the steps she chooses to take.

Sarah's story is one of many. Economic stability isn't about where you are today—it's about the direction you're moving in.

Practical Steps to Strengthen Economic Stability:

- **Expand Your Earning Potential with New Skills:** The world is full of opportunities to grow your income. No matter your current job or background, there are ways to build skills that open doors. Many community colleges, online platforms, and local organizations offer free or low-cost job training programs, career coaching, and certifications that can increase earning potential. Ask yourself: Is there a skill I've always been interested in learning that could create new opportunities? Whether it's digital marketing, healthcare support, coding, or a trade skill, investing in knowledge is investing in financial security.

- **Create a Simple Financial Snapshot:** Money feels overwhelming when we don't understand where it's going. Even writing down your income and biggest expenses can bring clarity. Start with one small habit—track your spending for one week. Not to cut everything out, but to see where you might have more choices than you realized. Financial clarity isn't about restriction; it's about understanding where you have power and making decisions that align with your goals.
- **Tap Into Financial Support and Guidance:** You don't have to figure it all out alone. Many nonprofit organizations, credit unions, and community programs offer financial counseling, debt management resources, and budgeting workshops. If saving is tough, look into community programs that help with food, rent, or childcare. These programs aren't just about survival—they can free up money so you can focus on long-term goals.
- **Build a Savings Habit—Even If It's Small:** Saving isn't about the amount; it's about the habit. If $100 a month feels impossible, start with $5. The act of setting something aside builds over time. Consider automating a small transfer to a savings account each payday. Even tiny amounts add up and create a buffer for unexpected situations.

- **View Financial Choices Through the Lens of Possibility:** Instead of seeing financial decisions only as sacrifices, try to see them as opportunities. For example, cooking at home instead of eating out could be viewed not just as "saving money" but as an opportunity to eat healthier or spend time with family. Taking on a side gig might not just be "more work" but a way to learn a new skill or meet new people.

(*Reflection:* Identify one financial habit you want to start, improve, or stop. How might this habit open up future possibilities for you?)

Education Access and Quality: Expanding Knowledge, Expanding Possibilities

Research from the National Bureau of Economic Research shows that people who engage in lifelong learning—whether through formal education or personal skill-building—experience greater job security, better health outcomes, and increased career fulfillment. The more we learn, the more we open doors for ourselves and others.

However, access to quality education isn't always easy. Some people grow up with strong support systems, mentors, and access to books, courses, and career training. Others might not—and that's okay, because it's never too late. Learning opportunities exist everywhere; sometimes we just need to know where to find them.

If you've ever felt like the educational resources available to you weren't enough, remember: opportunities for learning can often be found or created. Your story can always include a new chapter of growth.

Practical Steps to Strengthen Education Access and Personal Growth:

- **Take Advantage of Free or Low-Cost Online Classes:** Education has never been more accessible. Websites like Coursera, edX, and Khan Academy offer free or affordable courses on everything from business skills to creative writing to health sciences. Many public libraries also offer free online learning platforms and career development workshops. Is there something you've always wanted to learn more about? Now might be the time to explore it.
- **Find a Mentor or Join a Learning Community:** Personal growth is more manageable with someone to guide or encourage you. A mentor could be a teacher, a colleague, or someone in your network who has experience in an area you want to grow in. If mentorship feels out of reach, consider joining an online community, a local class, or a peer group focused on personal development. Learning often happens best when we're in conversation with others.
- **Utilize Local Educational Resources:** Libraries are a goldmine of free learning opportunities. From books to digital resources to language-learning apps, they offer tools many people overlook. Community centers, nonprofits, and adult learning programs often provide free skill-building courses, GED prep, and career counseling for those looking to expand their education. Make a list of resources in your area—you might be surprised what's available.

(*Reflection:* What's one topic, skill, or area of interest you've always wanted to explore? What's one step you can take to start learning about it today—signing up for a class, finding a book, or watching a tutorial?)

Seeing Education and Environment as Interconnected: Just as a strong neighborhood provides opportunities for connection, a strong educational foundation provides growth opportunities. For example, a safe, well-resourced community often has better access to schools, libraries, and adult learning programs. As knowledge increases, so do job opportunities and financial security, which can lead to improved living conditions. In turn, learning about community advocacy might give people tools to improve their communities. Growth in one area leads to growth in others. When you invest in your personal development, you're shaping your future and creating a ripple effect that touches those around you.

Your Next Step (Education): Think about how your physical space and ability to learn play roles in your life. Regardless of where you live or what resources you have now, you can always take steps to create more opportunities for yourself.

Ask yourself:

- How does my environment support or limit my well-being and learning?
- What learning opportunities excite me, and how can I start exploring them?
- What's one small action I can take today to improve the spaces I live in or expand my personal development?

Every bit of effort you put into building a stronger foundation—whether by improving your environment or deepening your education—is an investment in yourself and your future. And every step forward opens the door to even greater possibilities.

(*Remember:* Your surroundings and your education don't define you—they are tools that you can shape, adjust, and use to create the life you want. Strengthening one often helps strengthen the other.)

Food, Community, and Healthcare: Nourishing the Body, Mind, and Soul

If there's one universal truth, it's this: we all need nourishment—physically, socially, and emotionally. Food, community, and healthcare are deeply intertwined. Eating well gives us energy to engage with the world. When we feel connected socially, we have support to overcome challenges. When we have access to healthcare, we feel empowered to care for ourselves and those we love.

These areas of life aren't luxuries; they are essential foundations of well-being. Yet for many, access to healthy food, strong relationships, and quality healthcare can feel out of reach. If that's been your experience, know this: change is always possible. No matter where you start, there are ways to create small shifts that have lasting impact.

Let's explore how.

Food: Fueling Your Body and Your Future

Food isn't just fuel—it's connection, culture, and nourishment. It's a basic need that's deeply tied to how we experience life. Unfortunately, access to healthy food isn't equal for everyone. Financial constraints, food deserts, and time limitations can make eating well difficult. But no matter your situation, there are achievable ways to improve your relationship with food and make healthy eating a more realistic part of your life.

Practical Steps to Strengthen Food Access and Nutrition:

- **Identify Local Resources for Affordable, Nutritious Food:** Many communities have food banks, farmers' markets, or community gardens that provide fresh produce. Even if grocery stores are far, local organizations might offer food assistance or affordable meal programs. Websites like Feeding America can help you locate nearby food banks and meal services. Don't hesitate to make use of these resources—they exist to support you.
- **Plan Simple, Nutritious Meals with Affordable Ingredients:** Eating healthy doesn't have to be out of reach. Small changes, like adding more vegetables to meals and cutting back on processed foods, can make a difference. Try meal planning with budget-friendly staples that can be used in multiple dishes (beans, rice, eggs, frozen vegetables, etc.). If time is an issue, consider cooking in batches so you have meals ready for several days.
- **Join a Social Group Focused on Healthy Eating:** Food is often a source of connection. Try joining a community group, online forum, or class that shares healthy recipes, meal-planning tips, or cooking techniques. Some areas have nutrition programs or free/low-cost cooking classes that can help you learn

to prepare healthier meals. Sharing this journey with others can provide motivation and support.

(*Reflection:* What is one small change you can make this week to create a healthier and more enjoyable relationship with food? It could be trying one new healthy recipe, swapping a sugary drink for water, or eating fruit for a snack instead of chips.)

Community and Social Context: The Power of Belonging

Human beings are wired for connection. Studies from Harvard's Center on the Developing Child show that strong relationships are among the most important predictors of long-term health and happiness. Yet loneliness and isolation are more common than ever, leaving many people feeling disconnected.

The good news: building relationships doesn't have to be overwhelming. Small, intentional steps—reaching out to an old friend, joining a group, volunteering—can help you feel more connected and supported. (Volunteering, in particular, is a great way to meet like-minded people and feel the impact of making a difference.)

Practical Steps to Strengthen Community and Social Connection:

- **Volunteer with a Local Organization:** Giving back is one of the most powerful ways to connect with new, like-minded people. Websites like VolunteerMatch can help you find opportunities that match your interests. Whether it's helping at a food pantry, an animal shelter, or a literacy program, volunteering helps you make a positive impact in your community and meet others.

- **Rebuild Relationships One Step at a Time:** If you've lost touch with someone, set a small goal to reconnect this month. It can be as simple as a text, an email, a note, or a phone call. Often, people are happy to hear from you and pick up where you left off. Taking a few minutes to reach out can open the door to feeling close again.
- **Join a Club, Group, or Online Community:** Many community centers or libraries host free or low-cost events where you can meet people in a relaxed environment. Consider joining a book club, a fitness class, a faith community, or even an online forum related to a hobby. Meeting people with shared interests can quickly foster a sense of belonging.

(*Reflection:* What is one way you can strengthen your sense of connection with others this month? Maybe attend a local event, call a family member you haven't spoken to in a while, or introduce yourself to a neighbor you see regularly.)

Healthcare: Taking Charge of Your Well-Being

Navigating the healthcare system can feel overwhelming, especially when access is limited. But your health is worth advocating for. Studies from the National Institutes of Health show that people who feel comfortable communicating with their healthcare providers experience better health outcomes. This means that finding providers who listen to you, understanding your options, and feeling confident asking questions can make a real difference.

Practical Steps to Strengthen Your Healthcare Access and Experience:

- **Find Healthcare Resources That Fit Your Needs:** Healthcare can be intimidating, but it's possible to find access that works for you. Explore websites like NeedyMeds or the Health Resources and Services Administration (HRSA) site to locate low-cost medical services in your area. Many communities have free health screenings, clinics with sliding-scale fees, or programs to help with specific needs. Don't hesitate to think outside the box and look for creative solutions—sometimes a community health center or telehealth service can fill a gap.
- **Prepare for Medical Appointments with Confidence:** Many people feel nervous or rushed during medical appointments. You can take steps to feel more in control. Before your visit, write down your symptoms, medications, and any concerns. If you feel rushed or confused during the appointment, practice asking direct questions like, "Could you explain that in simpler terms?" or "What are my treatment options?"
- **Find Healthcare Providers Who Align with Your Needs:** Not every doctor or clinic will be the right fit for you. If you've ever felt misunderstood or not heard by a provider, know that you deserve better. Ask for referrals to providers who are culturally competent or who speak your primary language if that's a barrier. Many hospitals have patient advocacy programs—don't hesitate to reach out to them for help finding someone who meets your needs.

(Reflection: What is one small step you can take to feel more confident and empowered in managing your healthcare? For example, could you research a new clinic, prepare questions for your next appointment, or ask a friend to come with you as support?)

Bringing It All Together: Nourishing Every Part of Life

Food, community, and healthcare are deeply connected. When we nourish our bodies, we have more energy to engage with others. When we build strong relationships, we feel supported in our healthcare journeys. Taking charge of our health creates a foundation for a fuller, more vibrant life.

The path to strengthening these areas isn't about making massive changes all at once—it's about taking one small, meaningful step at a time.

As you reflect on your journey, ask yourself:

- What is one step I can take this week to improve my relationship with food?
- How can I build more meaningful connections in my life?
- What is one way I can feel more confident in navigating my healthcare?

Each of these steps is an investment in yourself—and in others. Your well-being matters, and every action, no matter how small, creates a ripple effect toward a healthier, more fulfilling life.

Each significant change truly begins with a single step.

Let's recall some of our earlier examples: Terry, Emma, Jonathan, Maria (from our case studies). They each faced barriers, but their lives began to change with one action: Terry found help getting her documents; Emma attended a nutrition workshop; Jonathan joined a veterans' group; Maria connected with a bilingual doctor. None of them solved everything overnight. They started with small steps, and those steps built momentum.

This is our nudge to take charge of our journey. There is power in movement. Change doesn't come from waiting for the perfect moment—it comes from choosing to take a step, no matter how small, and then taking another.

By strengthening your Social Determinants of Health, you're not trying to fix everything at once. You're choosing progress over perfection, one thoughtful decision at a time.

If you've made it this far in the toolkit, you've already started. You've reflected on where you are, gained insight into factors shaping your well-being, and identified areas for potential growth. Now the question is: **What will you do with this knowledge?**

Pause for a moment. Think about the stories you've read—the people who, despite barriers, found ways forward. Their lives didn't change overnight. Their transformations came from small, intentional choices that built momentum:

- Terry's first step toward economic stability was not achieving financial security overnight—it was finding someone to help her retrieve her missing documents.
- Emma's improvement in food security didn't start with perfect budgeting—it started with attending a single community workshop and food program.

- James (from our introduction) didn't wake up to a full pantry one day—his progress might begin by connecting with a local food co-op or community assistance program.

Their journeys were built one decision, one action, one moment of courage at a time.

The Power of Small Steps

Every significant change starts as something small. Consider the compounding effect of consistent actions:

These aren't grand or overwhelming commitments. They are small choices that, when repeated, lay the foundation for lasting change.

You Already Have What You Need to Begin. The capacity for change is within you. You've done hard things before—you've learned, adapted, cared for others, survived tough times. The skills and resilience that got you this far in life will serve you as you take on new challenges.

Remember: progress does not require perfection. It requires persistence, patience, and intentionality. Reflect on the goals you've set or the ideas you've had while reading this toolkit:

- What excites you most?
- What small action can you take today?
- If you're feeling unsure, that's okay—growth often starts with discomfort. But just by setting goals and reflecting, you are already moving forward.

The next step is to take action, one step at a time. Together, we can build a future where well-being is achievable.

SECTION 4

SOCIAL CARE – APPLYING SDOH IN YOUR WORK AND LIFE (PERSONALLY AND WITH OTHERS)

By this point, we turn our focus to an important movement called **Social Care**. You've reflected on your own life, uncovered strengths, and identified areas for growth. You've learned how to interpret your survey results, recognizing barriers that shaped your experiences and opportunities that can guide your next steps. You've seen how others navigated challenges, proving that change is possible and within reach. Most importantly, you now have actionable steps to build a roadmap toward a more stable, fulfilling, and empowered life.

Now, let's go deeper into the purpose of this whole approach—Social Care—which can be summarized as Everyone Seen. Everyone Heard.

We're in this together, and that's a very good thing. If you feel like you need more guidance, clarity, or simply someone to talk with who understands, we want you to reach out. (Visit tellegacy.org for resources, tools, and support, or connect directly with me at jeremyholloway.com.) Your growth is important, your journey matters, and we are here to walk alongside you as you take next steps.

Knowledge alone doesn't create change. Awareness of SDOH lays the foundation, but action transforms lives. A strong understanding of SDOH makes it possible to bridge the gap between reflection and real-world application related to health goals and actually achieving them—both individually and together.

A culture of social care values emotional and social well-being as much as physical health. It sees individuals in their full context—not just as patients, clients, or statistics, but as whole people navigating complex systems, relationships, and circumstances. This section explores ways to apply SDOH knowledge in daily life, strengthening your personal well-being while also making a broader impact.

Everyone Seen. Everyone Heard.

The Urgency of Social Care: A Vision for Change

Consider a world where no one has to choose between paying rent and buying medication. A world where a doctor asks about food security as routinely as checking blood pressure. A world where people feel connected and supported, no longer weighed down by isolation.

These shifts are not unattainable ideals. They happen when individuals, communities, and organizations integrate social care into everyday interactions.

For decades, healthcare and social services focused primarily on treating conditions, often overlooking the social and environmental forces that shape well-being. A report from the National Academy of Medicine estimates that up to 80% of health outcomes are influenced by social and economic factors rather than medical care alone. This means housing, education, employment, food access, and community support play as much of a role in health as medications and treatments.

Think about it: A prescription for high blood pressure may not help if fresh food isn't available in a person's neighborhood. A diabetes treatment plan is hard to follow if financial instability creates constant stress and uncertainty. Chronic conditions can worsen in the absence of strong social connections.

Addressing these factors leads to more equitable health outcomes, stronger communities, and improved quality of life. Social care is about preventing and treating the root causes of poor health, shifting focus from short-term fixes to long-term stability.

Shifting from Awareness to Action

The responsibility for improving SDOH doesn't rest solely on policymakers or healthcare leaders. Meaningful change happens through small, consistent actions—conversations with loved ones, interactions in professional settings, and how we share resources day-to-day.

Understanding and applying SDOH in daily life makes a difference, whether you're helping a client, a friend, a neighbor, or yourself.

A practical framework for integrating SDOH into personal and professional life can be broken into three key areas:

1. **Strengthening personal well-being**
2. **Supporting others in navigating challenges**
3. **Advocating for systemic change**

Each area plays a role in building a culture where social care and health equity are priorities.

Strengthening Personal Well-Being

Before guiding others, it's essential to recognize your own strengths and challenges. Well-being is an ongoing process that requires reflection, self-care, and access to support systems.

Self-assessment (like the one you did) helps identify areas that feel stable and areas that might need attention. Ask yourself questions like:

- How accessible are health services to me when I need them?
- Are my financial resources sufficient to cover basic needs without constant stress?
- Do I have a strong support network, personally and professionally?
- Are my educational or career goals aligned with my current circumstances?

Recognizing gaps isn't about self-judgment; it's about understanding where you might need extra support or action.

Building Support Networks: Thriving in any area of life doesn't have to be done in isolation. In fact, it often isn't. Seeking mentorship, forming relationships with like-minded people, and engaging with support groups all strengthen resilience. Having someone to turn to in moments of uncertainty can lighten the mental load and make barriers more manageable.

(If you feel like you don't have someone, remember that communities and professionals like us are here to connect with you.)

Advocating for Personal Needs: Systems can be hard to navigate, but together it's possible. Remember that advocating for yourself or a loved one often leads to better access to care, financial assistance, and social support. Whether in a medical appointment, at work, or with a landlord, asking direct questions and seeking clarity ensures you fully utilize available resources. Don't hesitate to speak up about what you need.

Supporting Others in Navigating Challenges

For those in healthcare, social work, case management, or caregiving roles, there is an opportunity to bridge the gap between systems and individuals. Many people face barriers they don't know how to overcome, and having a trusted guide can make all the difference.

Asking Meaningful Questions: Unless asked, many individuals won't volunteer information about financial hardship, housing insecurity, or food struggles. We need to normalize these discussions so people can share their experiences without shame or fear of judgment.

Instead of focusing solely on immediate issues, broaden the conversation with questions like:

- "What challenges are making daily life harder for you right now?"
- "Are there resources that could make things easier?"
- "Who or what provides the most support when things are difficult?"

A compassionate approach ensures people feel heard and valued, not just checked off on a form.

Becoming a Connector: No single person can change policies overnight or create large programs alone, but each of us can share knowledge and connect people to valuable resources. If you know of programs, share them.

- If someone lacks healthy food, tell them about local meal programs or a food pantry.
- If transportation is a barrier, mention subsidized transit passes or community ride services.
- If someone is lonely or dealing with mental health issues, suggest local activities or support groups.

You can't solve every problem, but you can open doors for people to access what they need. Small interventions—like telling someone about a resource—don't fix everything, but they create pathways that weren't there before.

Advocating for Systemic Change: Individual actions create meaningful improvements, but long-term change requires shifting how social care is prioritized at a structural level.

Imagine a healthcare system where:- Doctors routinely screen for social needs and refer patients to community resources.- Social workers have direct access to housing and employment support services for immediate solutions.- Community health workers are fully recognized as essential connectors, bridging clinical care with real-life needs.

These changes happen when communities, professionals, and policymakers collaborate to ensure well-being extends beyond clinic walls or social service offices.

Advocating for policy changes, supporting funding for social programs, and raising awareness of SDOH challenges can shift focus from treating crises to building stability.

The Collective Role in Creating Change: Whether you're working within a system, supporting a loved one, or reflecting on your own well-being, every action contributes to a broader movement. Building a culture of social care doesn't require grand gestures; it grows through small, intentional choices made every day.

By applying SDOH knowledge in meaningful ways—individually and collectively—we strengthen communities, expand opportunities, and make well-being a shared responsibility. The work doesn't fall on one person; real change becomes possible when many people take action together.

Using SDOH in Care Plans: Strategies for Caregivers, Social Workers, and CHWs

A care plan is more than a set of medical recommendations—it's a roadmap to well-being. When SDOH are integrated into care plans, the focus shifts from reactive treatment to proactive solutions, helping people thrive rather than just survive.

Care that considers social, economic, and environmental factors is more effective, more sustainable, and more human-centered. Instead of addressing the same issues repeatedly without lasting results, incorporating SDOH can break cycles of crisis by tackling root causes.

For caregivers, social workers, and community health workers, success lies in practical, achievable strategies. The goal isn't to overhaul entire systems overnight, but to weave

SDOH awareness into daily interactions through simple habits that compound over time.

Why SDOH Should Be Central to Care Plans: Traditional care models often address health challenges in isolation. For example, someone with chronic stress might receive anxiety medication but no support for their financial strain. A patient with diabetes might get nutrition advice without discussion of whether they can afford healthy food. This reactive approach leads to frustration, poor outcomes, and mistrust in the system.

When SDOH are at the center of care planning, everything changes. Trust is built, solutions are co-created, and outcomes improve because people feel truly seen.

Picture this: A case manager working with a client who has unstable housing doesn't just focus on medical treatment, but also connects them to housing resources, financial assistance, and mental health support. Or a social worker helping an elderly patient with limited mobility doesn't just arrange transport to doctor appointments, but also links them to community programs that reduce isolation.

The difference is profound: instead of just managing symptoms, we start transforming lives.

Making SDOH Practical in Everyday Care Plans:

Caregivers, CHWs, and social workers often don't have hours to redesign care plans from scratch. The key is to seamlessly incorporate SDOH assessments and interventions into existing workflows, using simple, repeatable habits.

- **Start with Open-Ended Questions:** How we frame questions matters. A yes/no question like "Do you have enough food?" might get a quick "yes" or "no" and miss the full picture. Shifting to open-ended prompts invites deeper insights:

- "Tell me about how you're managing meals right now."
- "What's your biggest challenge in making medical appointments?"
- "What's been feeling overwhelming lately?"

These small shifts allow people to share struggles without shame or defensiveness, leading to more accurate assessments and better care.

- **Normalize Conversations About SDOH:** Talking about housing, food security, finances, or social support can be hard, especially if someone has never been asked before. The way we introduce these topics can make someone feel comfortable or singled out. Normalize it by saying things like:
- "We ask everyone these questions because they matter so much to overall health."
- "Many people have challenges in these areas, and we want to make sure you have the support you need."

Presenting these discussions as a routine part of care strengthens trust and helps people feel less alone.

- **Document and Track Progress:** Consistency matters. Using simple SDOH checklists or notes can help track patterns, identify recurring challenges, and measure progress over time. Instead of documenting only medical updates, consider adding:
- housing stability check-ins

- food security assessments
- social connection updates (e.g., did the client join a support group or find someone to talk to?)

The goal isn't to drown in paperwork, but to integrate small, meaningful steps that build a fuller picture over time.

- **Collaborate with Clients on Solutions:** People are far more likely to engage with care plans when they feel ownership over them. As a caregiver or support person, your role isn't to dictate solutions but to co-create strategies with those you serve. Instead of saying, "You should apply for food assistance," try:
- "Would you be open to exploring local food resources together?"
- "Here are a few options we could look into—what do you think would work best for you?"

This shifts the focus from giving orders to fostering agency, making people active participants in their well-being.

Case Study: Applying SDOH in a Care Plan

Let's revisit Sarah's journey with diabetes and food insecurity. Sarah is 46 and struggles to manage her diabetes. She takes her medication, but her blood sugar remains unstable. In frustration, she tells her case manager that no matter what, she can't get her health under control.

Instead of immediately adjusting her medication, the case manager asks, "Tell me about how you're managing meals right now." Sarah hesitates, then admits she relies on fast food because it's the closest option. The nearest grocery store is over 5 miles away and she doesn't have a car.

Rather than giving generic nutrition advice, her case manager helps her identify a nearby food pantry that provides fresh produce. Together, they create a simple meal plan using ingredients from that pantry.

Within a few weeks, Sarah's blood sugar improves. More importantly, she feels heard, supported, and in control of her health for the first time.

Practical Ways to Strengthen SDOH Integration:

- **Create a Habit of Asking One SDOH-Related Question per Interaction:** Over time, this builds a fuller picture of needs without overwhelming conversations. For example, at each meeting or appointment, intentionally ask about one SDOH area (like housing or transportation). Rotate topics so you cover different areas over time.
- **Use the "One Small Action" Rule:** Every care plan should include one small, specific, achievable step related to SDOH. For example, instead of advising "improve food choices," reframe it as "visit the community food market this week and pick one new healthy item."
- **Celebrate Small Wins:** Recognizing small successes builds motivation and trust, making people more likely to stay engaged. For instance, if someone accessed a new resource for the first time, acknowledge that effort and success. ("I'm really glad you went to that community center—how did it go?")
- **Prioritize Relationships Over Checklists:** Care plans are useful tools, but human connection drives change. When people feel genuinely seen and

supported, they're far more likely to engage in their well-being. Don't let the process overshadow the person; the checklist should serve the relationship, not replace it.

A Future Built on Social Care

Care that embraces SDOH as a central pillar truly meets people where they are. It prevents crises before they escalate, strengthens relationships, and builds a system where people are supported holistically.

By shifting focus from isolated medical interventions to comprehensive social care, caregivers, CHWs, and social workers play a pivotal role in reshaping how we approach health and well-being.

Every question asked, every resource shared, every moment of connection moves us toward a healthier, more equitable future—one thoughtful step at a time.

Building Community Connections: The Power of Partnerships in Advancing Social Care

Social Determinants of Health are vast, complex, and interconnected. No single individual, organization, or sector can address them alone. The best outcomes arise when communities work together, leveraging resources, expertise, and shared goals to create sustainable change. Partnerships are the foundation of lasting impact—they create a web of support that improves access to resources, removes systemic barriers, and grows opportunities for individuals to thrive.

A report from the National Alliance to Impact the Social Determinants of Health (NASDOH) underscores this. Their research shows that cross-sector collaboration leads to better health outcomes, reduced healthcare costs, and improved community well-being. The ripple effect is profound when healthcare systems, local governments, social services, and community organizations align their efforts.

The key to success is intentionally building and maintaining relationships in the community so individuals and families receive the holistic support they need.

Why Community Partnerships Matter

Imagine the example of a single mother struggling to access healthcare because she doesn't have reliable transportation. She skips medical appointments, leading to worsening health conditions that could have been managed earlier. Now consider a healthcare provider who partners with a local transportation service to offer free or discounted rides to medical facilities. With that one connection, the mother gains consistent access to care, improving her health and reducing expensive emergency visits.

This is the power of community partnerships in action.

When organizations, agencies, and individuals unite with a shared mission, the impact goes beyond any single program or service. Healthcare access improves, food security strengthens, economic stability grows.

NASDOH's 2024 Year in Review highlights numerous case studies where multi-sector collaborations improved community health and well-being. One initiative paired financial literacy workshops with job training programs to provide families with economic stability. Another created community gardening projects in urban areas, improving access to fresh produce and strengthening social ties among neighbors.

These examples reinforce that no one can address SDOH alone, but together, real change is possible.

Steps to Build Meaningful Community Connections

Creating a network of support doesn't necessarily require massive funding or nationwide initiatives. It often begins with small, intentional steps at the local level—steps that caregivers, CHWs, social workers, and community advocates can take every day.

- **Start Locally:** Identify Key Organizations and Resources. Regardless of location, every community has organizations working on different SDOH issues. The key is finding them and figuring out how to collaborate. Essential organizations to connect with might include:
- Food security: local food banks, community gardens, nutrition programs.
- Healthcare access: free clinics, mobile health services, telehealth programs.
- Economic stability: workforce development centers, microloan organizations, financial counseling services.
- Housing and neighborhood: nonprofit housing groups, transportation services, neighborhood associations.
- Social and emotional support: peer support groups, volunteer organizations, senior centers.

Try attending community meetings, exploring local resource directories, and talking with community leaders.

Many organizations welcome partnerships and may already have referral programs in place.

- **Be Intentional:** Establish and Nurture Relationships. Partnerships aren't just about networking—they're about building trust and working toward shared goals. For professionals looking to integrate SDOH into care plans, this means:
- Reaching out with a clear purpose: Instead of a generic request, offer specific ways to collaborate. For example, "Our clinic works with families facing food insecurity; we'd like to explore a partnership to directly refer our patients to your food assistance services."
- Understanding each partner: Learn about the organization's mission, strengths, and challenges. Maybe a financial literacy nonprofit offers great workshops but struggles with outreach—by teaming up, both parties benefit (you get resources for your clients; they reach more people).
- Committing for the long-term: Trust takes time. Regular check-ins, joint events, and two-way referrals create sustainable partnerships that lead to real impact.

NASDOH's findings show that coalitions and long-term partnerships lead to bigger policy changes and funding for SDOH programs than one-off initiatives. Consistent engagement leads to more profound, lasting change.

- Stay Engaged: Strengthen the Web of Support. Once partnerships form, consistency is key. It's not enough to make a one-time referral or attend a single meeting; ongoing collaboration ensures resources remain accessible and relationships remain strong. Ways to stay engaged include:

- Attend community coalitions or interagency meetings regularly.
- Participate in joint outreach events (like health fairs or community days).
- Keep communication open—share updates, successes, and needs with partners.

A successful example comes from a city-wide initiative highlighted in NASDOH's report. Healthcare providers, housing services, and job training programs created a wraparound care model for people experiencing homelessness. Because these organizations stayed engaged and communicated often, individuals received coordinated care addressing immediate needs (like shelter) and long-term solutions (like employment and health services). The result: better outcomes all around.

The Impact of Collaboration: A Case Study

Bridging the Gap Between Healthcare and Housing

In 2022, a partnership between a hospital system and a nonprofit housing organization transformed care for patients facing chronic illness and housing instability.

The problem: Many patients with diabetes and heart disease kept landing in the hospital partly because they lacked stable housing and proper nutrition.

The solution: Healthcare providers partnered with a housing organization to offer temporary stable housing to high-risk patients, along with nutrition counseling and connections to community food programs.

The result: Within one year, hospital readmissions dropped by 40%. Patients reported improved mental health and better control of their chronic conditions. The collaboration even secured funding to expand the program to additional neighborhoods.

This initiative underscored the power of collaboration—where healthcare, housing, and food security intersect, lives can change.

The Future of Community Collaboration in SDOH

NASDOH's Proposed Principles for SDOH Research and Call to Action (2023) emphasized that the future of SDOH lies in collective action. Sustainable solutions need public-private partnerships, cross-sector collaboration, and innovative approaches.

Governments, healthcare institutions, nonprofits, and businesses all have roles in shaping health equity. But the most important work happens on the ground, in communities, through authentic relationships.

By strengthening partnerships, social workers, CHWs, caregivers, and community leaders create a future where health and well-being are accessible to all—as a right, not a privilege.

Building community connections doesn't just solve individual problems; it creates a culture of care that lasts generations.

Advocacy and Policy: Becoming a Voice for Change

The Power of Advocacy in Advancing SDOH

Addressing Social Determinants of Health takes more than individual actions or isolated programs. While direct interventions—like providing food assistance or free health screenings—are vital, lasting change comes when systems evolve to remove barriers and expand opportunities. This is where advocacy becomes critical.

Advocacy is the bridge between grassroots experiences and systemic change. It transforms individual struggles into policy reforms, funding increases, and institutional shifts that make resources more accessible and sustainable. For example, the work of Healthy People 2030 illustrates how policy-driven initiatives have made measurable strides in reducing poverty, increasing healthcare access, and improving public health standards.

However, advocacy isn't just for policymakers in suits—it's for anyone who cares about these issues. Whether you're a caregiver, a social worker, a CHW, or an engaged community member, you can be an advocate.

Why Advocacy Matters in SDOH

Imagine a community where people regularly face food insecurity because the nearest grocery store is miles away. Residents struggle with chronic illnesses that could be better managed with proper nutrition, yet no policies encourage grocery retailers to expand into these "food deserts."

Now, picture a group of local advocates stepping in—health professionals, social workers, community leaders—coming together to make their case to the city council. They bring data, share personal stories, and propose solutions, like tax incentives for grocery stores to open in underserved areas.

Within a year, their advocacy yields positive change: a new grocery store breaks ground, mobile produce markets are funded, or transportation options to better food outlets are improved. An entire neighborhood starts to feel the difference.

This is the power of advocacy—moving from temporary relief to lasting, scalable solutions.

How Policy Shapes SDOH

According to Healthy People 2030, significant progress in areas like healthcare access, economic stability, and education has often come from targeted policy interventions. Here are some examples:

- **Public Health Accreditation:** More state and local public health agencies have become accredited, improving health service standards nationwide (Healthy People PHI objectives).
- **Economic Stability Improvements:** The proportion of people living in poverty has begun to decline, and employment among working-age individuals has increased (SDOH objectives).
- **Healthcare Access Progress:** Fewer people are unable to get medical or dental care when needed (Healthcare Access objectives).
- **Youth Mental Health:** More adolescents are receiving treatment for depression, a result of increased mental health awareness and funding (Mental Health objectives).

These shifts didn't happen by accident—they resulted from years of persistent advocacy, policy changes, and strategic funding.

How to Become an Advocate for Change

Advocacy doesn't require a title or formal training—it requires commitment, persistence, and strategic action. Here are practical ways individuals can engage in advocacy at any experience level:

- **Share Stories that Bring SDOH to Life:** Data is important, but personal stories inspire action. Policymakers and decision-makers are more likely to support an initiative when they understand its human impact. For example, a social worker advocating for transportation services for the elderly might share the story of Ms. Rodriguez, an 82-year-old who missed medical appointments due to unreliable transit, leading to a preventable hospital admission. Pairing data with Ms. Rodriguez's story makes a compelling case, perhaps securing funding for a senior ride-share program.

How to do this: Collect real-life stories to share with policymakers, community leaders, and funders. If privacy is a concern, ask clients or community members to speak for themselves at public meetings or submit written testimony about how social factors affect them. Use social media, community forums, or newsletters to highlight success stories of how small changes (like a new bus route or a community garden) made a big difference.

- **Engage Locally and Use Your Voice in the Community:** Advocacy often starts local. Small policy changes at the city or county level can have immediate impact. For example, a group of nurses, social workers, and volunteers might see an increase in food insecurity after a factory closure. Instead of only waiting for federal aid, they attend town hall meetings, start petitions, and meet with city officials to expand local food assistance. Within months, the city funds mobile grocery markets, ensuring families get fresh food without traveling far.

Ways to engage locally: Attend city council or town hall meetings and speak during public comment. Partner with local organizations or coalitions already working on issues you care about. Write letters or request meetings with local officials to present community data and personal stories. Sometimes your voice can spark immediate action.

- **Leverage Networks and Collaborate for Greater Impact:** Advocacy is stronger when done collectively. Collaboration amplifies voices, adds credibility, and builds a movement for change. For example, a coalition of CHWs and social service organizations may see families struggling due to a lack of affordable housing. By aligning their efforts, they could launch a city-wide campaign for more affordable housing initiatives—maybe public forums, joint letters, and working with media. Together, they might achieve what one group alone couldn't: increased funding for rental assistance, new housing developments, or stronger tenant protections.

How to collaborate effectively: Join or form advocacy groups focused on SDOH (maybe a health equity task force or housing coalition). Partner with nonprofits, businesses, and healthcare systems that share your goals. Organize community awareness events to educate the public and gather support. The idea is that one person can make a difference, but many people working together can drive sweeping change.

Advocacy in Action: A Success Story

Fighting Food Insecurity Through Policy Change

A city had high rates of food insecurity, especially in low-income neighborhoods. Social workers and community health leaders noticed many families had no nearby grocery stores, relying instead on gas stations and convenience stores for food.

Instead of relying only on food pantries or short-term aid, advocates pushed for systemic changes: - They partnered with local farmers to create a subsidized farmers' market program.- They lobbied city officials to fund incentives attracting grocery stores to underserved areas.- They worked with state legislators to expand SNAP benefits to cover healthy meal delivery services.

Within two years, food insecurity was cut in half in the targeted neighborhoods. Children had better access to fresh fruits and vegetables, chronic disease rates declined, and overall community well-being improved.

This shows how advocacy can go beyond temporary help to create lasting, structural solutions.

Taking the First Step Toward Advocacy

Systemic change doesn't happen overnight, but every voice matters. The efforts of one advocate, one conversation, one policy at a time all contribute to a future where health isn't determined by ZIP code, income, or circumstance.

Advocacy isn't about knowing everything—it's about showing up. Whether through sharing a story, engaging in a community meeting, or collaborating with others, every action brings us closer to a world where health and well-being are accessible to all.

Now is the time to step forward, speak up, and make a difference—because real change begins when people decide that the barriers we've discussed are meant to be broken.

SECTION 5

WORKBOOK EXERCISES – SOLIDIFYING LEARNING AND TAKING ACTION

By now, the concepts around Social Determinants of Health are no longer abstract ideas. Through the previous sections, we have seen them take shape in personal experiences and stories of transformation. We've recognized how deeply health is connected to environment, relationships, and opportunities. But understanding is just the beginning.

Real transformation happens when knowledge turns into action—when we move from recognizing barriers to actively breaking them down. The most powerful change often doesn't start in government offices or grand movements; it begins with everyday choices. It begins right here.

This section is an invitation: to take everything you've learned and apply it to make a real, meaningful impact in your own life, your work, and your community.

Small Steps

Motivational speaker Lisa Nichols often explains that transformation isn't about massive, sweeping changes—it's about small, consistent steps taken with intention. Research professor Brené Brown reminds us that vulnerability is at the heart of real growth. These lessons apply to SDOH too.

No one has to solve everything overnight.

Strengthening SDOH—whether for yourself or those you serve—requires taking one step at a time with purpose and persistence.

So, let's begin by choosing a starting point, rather than feeling overwhelmed by everything that could be done. Every conversation that acknowledges a need can open space for a solution. Every connection to a resource can change a life. Every act of advocacy can contribute to a future where opportunity meets support.

Workbook Exercise 1: Self-Reflection – Finding Your SDOH Focus

Before jumping into action, it's important to pause and reflect. What area of SDOH matters most to you right now?

Consider the seven areas of SDOH—economic stability, education, healthcare access, neighborhood, social connections, food security, and work/recreation.

Take a moment to think about which one resonates most with your personal or professional experience at this moment.

Ask yourself:

- Which area of SDOH has affected my life the most?
- What challenges have I or people I care for faced in this area?
- Which area do I feel most drawn to work on improving?

(Write your reflections below. Be honest and open,

and most importantly, be kind to yourself. This isn't about judgment—it's about clarity.)

Your Reflection: - Focus *Area: [e.g., Healthcare Access]- Why it matters to me: [e.g., "I've seen family members struggle to get appointments and medication due to cost, and it's frustrating."]*

(You might list experiences or feelings—e.g., "I worry about my aging parents skipping check-ups because of distance to the clinic," or "I struggled with food insecurity in college and know how distracting and stressful that was.")

Workbook Exercise 2: Goal-Setting for Impact

Now that you've identified an area that matters most to you, it's time to create a real, actionable goal.

We will start small—because small, consistent actions lead to big change.

Think of something practical and achievable in the next 30 days related to your focus area.

Example Goals: - If you identified economic stability as your focus: "I will explore one financial literacy program and share the resource with someone who could benefit."- If you chose social connection: "I will reach out to an old friend or family member to strengthen my support system."- If your focus is healthcare access: "I will find a local free clinic or telehealth service and share that information with my community (or use it myself)."

Now, take a moment to write down your goal. Keep it simple and specific.

- **My Goal:** [Write a single sentence goal here]
- **Why this matters to me:** [Write a brief reason—this helps remind you of your motivation]

(For example: "My goal is to arrange transportation for my neighbor to get to her doctor appointment next week. This matters to me because I've seen her cancel visits due to lack of a ride, and I want her to get the care she needs.")

Workbook Exercise 3: Scenario-Based Practice – Applying SDOH in Real Life

Understanding SDOH conceptually is one thing, but applying it in everyday interactions is another. This exercise bridges that gap by using scenarios.

Scenario:

Imagine you are working with a client or helping a friend who is struggling with an SDOH-related barrier. They have opened up to you about a challenge, and you want to support them meaningfully.

Consider this situation:

Anna is a single mother who recently lost her job. She confides that she's behind on rent and worried about losing her apartment. She's never applied for housing assistance and doesn't know where to start.

Reflection Questions:

- What are the first three steps you could take to help Anna navigate this situation?
- What resources or local programs might be useful for her?
- How can you offer support while also empowering Anna to take action herself?

(Take a few minutes to jot down your thoughts. Think of concrete actions: e.g., help her search for emergency rental assistance

programs, connect her with a housing counselor, etc. Also consider how to involve Anna in these steps so she feels in control.)

Your Possible Approach for Anna:

Step 1: [e.g., "Listen to Anna's situation fully and reassure her she's not alone. Then help her prioritize immediate needs (rent, utilities)."]

Step 2: [e.g., "Research local housing assistance programs (city's emergency fund, charities like Salvation Army) and help her contact one."]

Step 3: [e.g., "Help Anna fill out a housing assistance application, or accompany her to a community center where she can apply. Encourage her to talk to her landlord about the situation if appropriate."]

Resources: [e.g., "2-1-1 hotline, local social services office for rent assistance, a church community program."]5. Empowerment: [e.g., "Explain each step so Anna can do these things on her own next time if needed. Provide her with a list of resources and contacts we found. Encourage her strengths (managing family, seeking help shows responsibility)."]

(This is just one scenario. You can practice with others: maybe someone facing food insecurity or someone feeling isolated. The idea is to apply what you know to real-world support.)

Workbook Exercise 4: Your Personal Action Plan – Making an Impact Beyond This Book

Knowledge becomes powerful when paired with ongoing commitment. This exercise helps you create an action plan that extends beyond today.

Long-Term Commitment to Change:

Think about how you want to continue making a difference beyond today: - How will you integrate SDOH awareness into your daily life or work?- How can you be more intentional in helping others navigate social needs?- What long-term impact do you hope to create?

Mapping Out Your Plan:

Fill in the following prompts:

- **A Habit I Want to Build Around SDOH Awareness:**
  Example: "I will ask my patients about their social needs in every consultation and provide at least one resource if needed."

  Your Habit: "I will ... [describe the habit]."

- **A Community Connection I Want to Strengthen:**
  Example: "I will attend a monthly community coalition meeting to better understand local resources."

  Your Plan: "I will ... [describe how you'll engage with a community or organization]."

- **A System I Want to Advocate For:**
  Example: "I will write to my local representatives about increasing access to mental health support in underserved areas."

  Your Advocacy Plan: "I will ... [describe one advocacy step, like writing a letter or joining an advocacy group]."

  (These commitments don't have to be overwhelming—they just need to be consistent. For instance, a habit could be as simple as spending 5 minutes each week learning about a new resource, or checking in on a neighbor regularly.)

Call to Action: Embracing a Culture of Social Care

No one moves forward alone. Health and well-being are built in connection, community, and daily choices.

Imagine a world where everyone has what they need to thrive—where support isn't a privilege but the standard. That world starts with the actions we take today.

Whether you are a caregiver, a healthcare provider, a social worker, or someone who just wants to make a difference, you have the power to create change.

The choice to advocate, support, and show up matters.

So take this moment: write down your goal, reach out to a resource, commit to a small action.

Because when small steps become daily habits, and daily habits grow into a culture, real transformation begins.

Turning Awareness into Achievable Steps: Goal-Setting Worksheets for Strengthening SDOH

Transformation doesn't happen by accident. It unfolds through intention, commitment, and small, deliberate steps that build toward something greater. This section is designed to move beyond awareness into application. By setting specific, measurable goals, we create momentum for lasting change, whether for personal growth or in helping others navigate their SDOH challenges. When we commit to real, tangible actions, we bridge the gap between where we are and where we want to be.

The beauty of small, consistent actions is that they lead to significant transformations over time. Whether you're aiming to improve your own stability or support someone else's journey, every intentional step counts.

Why Goal-Setting Matters in SDOH:

Big changes rarely happen in one day. They start with small, specific decisions that are realistic, achievable, and fit a person's life circumstances.

Behavioral research (like Dr. Edwin Locke's Goal-Setting Theory) emphasizes that clarity, challenge, commitment, and feedback are essential for successful goal achievement. Vague or overwhelming goals often get abandoned, whereas specific and actionable goals create motivation and accountability. Additionally, author James Clear (in Atomic Habits) shares that success comes from small, repeated behaviors that compound over time. Instead of chasing drastic, unsustainable change, focus on what can be improved today.

With these principles in mind, the following prompts will help you identify one achievable, measurable goal for each SDOH category you want to work on. These goals should be specific enough to be actionable and small enough to create momentum.

Setting Personal and Professional Goals for SDOH:

For each category you want to address, choose at least one goal (personal or to support someone else). Write it down, commit to it, and visualize the impact.

Economic Stability: Creating Financial

SecurityReflection: What's one step you can take in the next six months to improve financial health or reduce financial stress?Example Goals:- Apply for one local job training program that aligns with your career goals (this week).- Meet with a financial counselor to create a budget and identify savings strategies (in the next two weeks).- Research local small business grants or microloans for a business idea (within the next month).– Set up an emergency savings account and commit to adding a small amount each month.

Write Your Goal: [Your specific goal related to economic stability]

- **Neighborhood and Physical Environment:** Building a Supportive SpaceWhere we live and the resources available in our community greatly influence our health and well-being.Reflection: How can you make your living environment more supportive of well-being?Example Goals:– Attend one local neighborhood meeting to advocate for a community need (safer streets, better transit, etc.).– Join a local community advocacy group focused on housing or environmental improvements.– Improve your home environment by creating a peaceful, organized space for relaxation or work.– Find a safe outdoor area and commit to walking or exercising there regularly.

Write Your Goal: *[Your specific goal related to neighborhood/ environment]*

- **Education Access and Quality:** Investing in Lifelong LearningEducation opens doors, whether through formal schooling, self-directed learning, or skill-building. Continued learning fuels success and empowerment.Reflection: What's one way you can invest in personal or professional growth?Example Goals:– Enroll in a free or low-cost online course on a topic of interest (this month).– Sign up for a workshop that could improve your career skills (next available date).– Get involved in a mentorship program, as either a mentor or mentee, in the next quarter.– Visit a library or community center to explore learning resources (this week).

Write Your Goal: *[Your specific goal related to education]*

- **Food Security:** Ensuring Access to Nutritious FoodFood is fundamental to mental, physical, and emotional health. Reliable access to nutritious food reduces stress and improves overall well-being. Reflection: What's one step you can take to improve access to nutritious food?Example Goals:- Find and visit a local farmers' market or food pantry (this week).- Set up a meal-planning system that includes affordable, healthy foods (this month).- Learn one new healthy recipe each week and cook at home more often.- Start a small herb or vegetable garden (even a windowsill garden) to have fresh ingredients.

Write Your Goal: *[Your specific goal related to food security]*

- **Community and Social Context:** Strengthening Meaningful ConnectionsRelationships shape our resilience and mental health. Feeling seen and supported is crucial for life satisfaction.Reflection: What's one way you can strengthen your connection to others?Example Goals:- Attend one community event or volunteer opportunity this month to meet new people.- Set up a recurring check-in (weekly or monthly) with a friend, neighbor, or family member.- Join a local group or online forum centered on a hobby or interest.- Participate in a support group focused on personal growth or a challenge you're facing.

Write Your Goal: *[Your specific goal related to social connections]*

- **Healthcare Access and Quality:** Taking Charge of Well-BeingQuality healthcare isn't just about having insurance; it's about navigating the system, advocating for your needs, and getting care that works for you.Reflection: What's one step you can take to ensure your healthcare needs are met?Example Goals:– Schedule a wellness check-up with a trusted provider (this month).– Research clinics that offer sliding-scale fees or free services and share with someone who needs it (this week).– Prepare a list of questions before your next doctor's appointment to feel more confident and get the info you need.– Look for healthcare providers that align with your values (e.g., those who speak your language or specialize in your needs) and make a plan to transition if necessary.

Write Your Goal: *[Your specific goal related to healthcare]*

(For each goal above, ensure it's something you can reasonably do. The idea is to commit to it, track progress, and adjust as needed. Write these goals on a paper or digital notepad you see often.)

Encouragement and Final Thoughts: The Power of Commitment

Committing to change—even in small ways—creates a ripple effect that extends far beyond individual actions.

Progress doesn't require perfection. It requires persistence, patience, and intentionality.

Take a moment to reflect on the goals you've written: - What excites you most about these plans?- What challenges might come up, and how could you address them?- How do you envision feeling as you make progress in these areas?

Remember, feeling unsure or uncomfortable is okay. Growth often starts with some discomfort. But the fact that you've set these goals means you are already moving forward.

The next step is action—one step at a time. Together, we can build a future where well-being is within reach.

(By now, you have practical steps and goals to carry forward. Refer back to these exercises regularly. Celebrate the small wins, adjust your strategies as needed, and never hesitate to seek support or resources. You are part of a community that cares, and your efforts—big or small—contribute to a larger movement for health equity and social care.)

CASE STUDIES

Let's look at some real-world examples to see how these principles come together. These case studies illustrate the challenges and triumphs of people addressing SDOH in their lives. As you read, note what actions made a difference and think about how similar approaches might apply in your context.

Case Study 1: Breaking the Cycle – Terry's Journey to Economic Stability

Terry was 22, standing at the threshold of adulthood, yet every door seemed locked. She grew up surrounded by instability—poverty and dysfunction were her earliest memories. Her father was in and out of prison before disappearing entirely. Her mother, battling addiction, was physically present but not emotionally available.

When Terry's mother could no longer care for her, Terry's older sister took legal custody. That should have been a turning point—someone to guide and protect her as she transitioned to independence. Instead, it became another roadblock. For reasons Terry never understood, her sister refused to give her access to critical documents (birth certificate, Social Security card). Without those, Terry couldn't get a driver's license, apply for jobs, or enroll in assistance programs.

She was trapped by bureaucracy: she needed proof of identity to gain access to opportunity, but she couldn't obtain that proof on her own. Every attempt met the same answer: "Come back when you have your paperwork." It felt like the world didn't recognize her as a person.

Then she found Project Ascend, a program at a local youth clinic designed to help young people like her—those left behind by the system but determined to change their trajectory. At first, Terry was skeptical; she had learned not to trust promises of help. But Project Ascend was different.

The program connected her to healthcare services she'd never had. She had struggled with headaches and blurry vision for years but never had a proper eye exam. Project Ascend set her up with an optometrist, and she finally got glasses. The clarity was more than just literal vision; it was the realization that she deserved basic care and resources.

Healthcare was just the beginning. A counselor at the clinic saw Terry's potential and encouraged her to enroll in an EKG technician certification course at the community college. The program was fully funded—an opportunity she couldn't have afforded on her own. For the first time, she had a structured path toward a stable career.

Even as she excelled in her coursework, another shadow loomed: housing insecurity. Without stable housing, finishing her certification and finding work would be an uphill battle. Recognizing this, Project Ascend stepped in again, securing donations to cover a few months' rent for her. That stability allowed her to focus, study, and plan her future without the constant stress of wondering where she'd sleep.

Perhaps the most transformative moment came when program staff helped her retrieve her missing documents. After years of feeling invisible, she finally had the papers needed to apply for jobs, open a bank account, and become independent.

By the time Terry completed her certification, she had also secured part-time work to support herself. It wasn't just about the paycheck; it was about building a future. She had spent years feeling stuck while watching others move forward. Now she was in motion.

Key Lesson: Economic stability is often seen as a financial issue, but Terry's story shows it's about access and removing barriers. Money was part of it, but even more, it was about having documentation, mentorship, and programs that provided tangible support. It took mentors who saw her potential, programs that offered real help (not just advice), and systems that made success possible. For Terry, economic stability meant reclaiming her identity, building a career, and most importantly, believing in a future that once felt out of reach.

Case Study 2: Overcoming Food Insecurity Through Community Support

Emma, a single mother of two, worked full-time but struggled to make ends meet. Despite careful budgeting, she often had to choose between paying rent and buying nutritious food.

She lived in a food desert—a neighborhood with limited access to fresh produce and healthy meals. The nearest full grocery store was miles away. Without reliable transportation, fast food and convenience store options became the default.

Feeling overwhelmed, Emma reached out to a community food program aimed at helping working families. Through this program, she started going to a local food bank that distributed fresh produce each week. She also enrolled in a nutritional workshop where she learned to cook healthy meals on a budget. Additionally, Emma joined a community meal-sharing group—families in her area took turns preparing and delivering home-cooked meals to each other on a schedule.

Transformation and Outcome: Within a few months, Emma spent less on food while actually eating healthier. Her children's energy improved; she no longer had to skip meals to ensure they were fed. The community connections she built through the meal-sharing program also became a source of emotional support, reducing her stress levels.

Key Lesson: Food insecurity isn't just about finances—it's about access, education, and community-driven solutions that empower people to take control of their health. Emma's story shows that when given access to resources (food bank produce), knowledge (cooking classes), and community support (meal-sharing and emotional encouragement), families can break the cycle of unhealthy eating and insecurity.

Case Study 3: Rebuilding Social Connections for Mental and Emotional Well-Being

Jonathan, a 54-year-old retired military veteran, had spent his life moving from city to city. After his last relocation to a new city where he knew almost no one, he felt isolated and disconnected.

Without strong social ties, Jonathan's mental health started to decline. He experienced depression and anxiety but hesitated to seek help. His turning point came when he visited a veteran resource center. A social worker there encouraged him to join a local veterans' group so he could connect with others who shared similar experiences.

Jonathan took the advice and also found a volunteer mentorship program where he could guide younger veterans transitioning into civilian life. This mentorship gave him a renewed sense of purpose. He also started attending weekly meet-ups at a community center focused on veterans' social activities and personal growth workshops.

Transformation and Outcome: Jonathan regained a sense of purpose and belonging as he rebuilt his social network. His mental health improved significantly. He eventually became an advocate at the resource center, reaching out to other veterans facing loneliness and isolation, encouraging them to connect like he did.

Key Lesson: Social connections are a fundamental determinant of health. Finding a supportive community—even in unexpected places—can provide emotional resilience and improve mental well-being. Jonathan's willingness to engage (with some encouragement) not only improved his health but also positioned him to help others.

Case Study 4: Navigating the Healthcare System with Confidence

Maria, a 37-year-old immigrant, faced several barriers to healthcare. She spoke limited English and struggled to communicate her needs during medical appointments. Even though she qualified for low-cost health services, she avoided going to the doctor due to language barriers and past experiences of not being taken seriously.

Her breakthrough came when a bilingual patient advocate at a community clinic helped her find a culturally competent physician who spoke her preferred language. This advocate also taught Maria how to prepare for appointments—writing down her symptoms and questions beforehand—and connected her to a sliding-scale clinic for affordable follow-up treatments.

Transformation and Outcome: With these changes, Maria felt empowered to seek medical care without fear. She addressed health concerns that had been lingering for years. By learning how to navigate the system and finding providers she could trust, she became proactive in managing her health.

Key Lesson: Healthcare access isn't just about availability—it's about cultural competence, trust, and equipping patients with tools to navigate the system confidently. Maria's story underlines that addressing language and trust barriers can transform someone from avoiding care to actively engaging in their health.

Bringing It All Together: The Power of Holistic Support

Each case highlights a crucial truth: No single factor operates in isolation.

- Economic stability leads to better healthcare, food, and housing options.
- Food security impacts physical and emotional health, reducing stress and boosting productivity.
- Social connections provide mental resilience and emotional strength.
- Accessible healthcare ensures individuals can

maintain and improve their quality of life.

When we address SDOH as interconnected pieces of a larger puzzle, we move beyond temporary fixes and create long-term pathways to success.

Your Next Step: Reflecting on Your Own Story

After reading these stories, take a moment to reflect on your own situation: - What barriers have you faced, and what strengths helped you overcome them?- Which area of your well-being (economic, social, health, etc.) needs the most support right now?- Who or what in your community could be a resource for your personal growth?

Transformation is not solely about where you start; it's about the steps you take. No matter where you are in your journey, change is always possible.

Let these stories remind you that every challenge carries an opportunity, every barrier can be navigated, and every person has the capacity for growth.

Your Roadmap to Strengthen Social Determinants of Health

Now that we've explored how SDOH shape our well-being, let's bring the focus back to you. Reflection is valuable, but action creates real change. Small steps can shift your trajectory no matter where you're starting from. The following exercise is designed to help you take one intentional step toward strengthening an area of your life—not through overwhelming change, but through focused, achievable action.

- **Step One:** Choose One Area to Focus OnThink about the different SDOH areas: economic stability, education, healthcare access, neighborhood, social connections, food and nutrition, work and recreation. Which one stands out as having the most potential for growth for you right now?Perhaps you're financially strained and want to work toward stability. Maybe your social circle has changed and you want deeper connections. Or you've been putting off healthcare and want to change that.There's no wrong choice. The goal isn't to "fix" everything—it's to start where you are and move forward intentionally.Which area of your life would benefit most from focused attention? Write it down or say it out loud to acknowledge it.

- **Step Two:** Set One Actionable GoalNow that you've picked a focus, define one clear, specific goal to move forward. Make it small enough to be achievable but meaningful enough to build momentum.If your focus is finances, a focused goal might be: "Create a simple budget this week to track my spending."If it's health: "Schedule a check-up with a provider I trust this month."If it's social: "Attend one community event or call one friend this week."This isn't about a "perfect" goal, just one step in the direction you want to go.Write down one goal that is specific, actionable, and realistic for the next week or month.
- **Step Three:** Identify Your ResourcesGoals become easier when we have the right tools or people supporting us. Consider what resources are available to help you move forward.If your goal is career-related, maybe the local library has free resume workshops.If it's health, perhaps there's a community clinic or an app for scheduling appointments.If it's diet, maybe

you have a friend who's great at meal prepping who could share tips.Who or what can support you in reaching your goal? Write down at least one resource (a website, a book, a mentor, a community program, a friend or family member, etc.).

- **Step Four:** Take One Immediate ActionMomentum builds by doing something right away—today, if possible. When you take even a tiny step, you start to create progress.If your goal is to find a new job, one immediate step could be to spend 10 minutes today searching for job openings or updating your resume. If your goal is to meet people, you could text an old friend right now or look up a local meetup group.If your goal is health-related, you might call the doctor's office or go for a short walk today.The action doesn't have to be big—it just has to be something you can do now.What is one thing you can do today to move toward your goal? Write it down and then do it.

(This exercise isn't about fixing everything overnight. It's about recognizing that you can create movement in your life. Change doesn't wait for the "perfect" moment or all the answers—it comes from choosing one step, then another.)

Remember: wherever you are today is not where you have to stay. This is your roadmap. And the best part? The next step is entirely yours to take.

Call to Action: Take Charge of Your Journey

There is power in movement. Change doesn't happen by waiting for the right moment—it happens by deciding to take a step, no matter how small, and then taking another. Strengthening your SDOH isn't about fixing everything at once. It's about choosing progress over perfection, one intentional decision at a time.

If you've come this far, you've already started. You've reflected on where you stand, gained insight into factors shaping your well-being, and identified areas for growth. Now, the question is: What will you do with this knowledge?

Pause and consider: Think about the stories of Terry, Emma, Jonathan, and Maria. Despite their barriers, each found a way forward. Their lives didn't change overnight or through giant leaps. Their transformations began with small, intentional choices that gained momentum: - Terry's journey to financial stability began by getting help with lost documents—one step that opened many doors.- Emma's improvements in health started by attending a nutrition class—one meeting that changed how she fed her family.- Jonathan's new purpose came from joining a weekly meetup—one social outing that combated years of isolation.- Maria's empowerment started with meeting one patient advocate—one conversation that changed her healthcare experience.

Their journeys were built one decision, one action, one moment of courage at a time.

The Hardest Part of Any Journey is Starting. But here's a truth: You've already started.

The Power of Small Steps: Every big change begins as a small one. Consider how consistent small actions can add up: - One extra glass of water a day -> better hydration over time.- 10 minutes learning a new skill daily -> new knowledge and opportunities.- Reaching out to one friend a week -> a stronger support network.- 5 minutes of walking each day

-> improved mobility and health.- Saving $5 each week -> an emergency fund for unexpected needs.

These aren't dramatic actions. They're simple, sustainable choices that, repeated over time, build the foundation for significant change.

You Are Already Equipped to Begin. You've overcome challenges before. You've learned new things, adapted to new circumstances, helped others, and survived difficulties. The resilience and skills that got you this far will help you in the steps ahead.

Remember: - Progress requires persistence, not perfection.- Every step, even if it seems small or imperfect, is movement forward.- It's okay if some days feel like setbacks—use them as learning, not as reasons to stop.

Think about the goals you set earlier: - Which one are you most excited about?- What small action can you do today to honor that excitement?- If doubts or obstacles come up, how will you remind yourself why this matters?

If you're feeling unsure or a bit overwhelmed, that's normal. Growth often feels that way at first. But by setting goals and planning steps, you've already activated change.

Next Steps: - Take that immediate action you identified—do it today if you can.- Keep this toolkit or your notes somewhere visible. Review your goals and progress regularly (daily or weekly).- Celebrate the small wins. Did you make that phone call? Meet that person? Save that money? Acknowledge it.- Adjust if necessary. If something isn't working, tweak your plan but keep moving. Ask for help or more resources if you need them.

We're in This Together: As you take each step, remember you're not doing it alone. There are communities, professionals, friends, and family who can and will support you if you reach out. You are also part of a larger movement of people striving to improve their lives and the lives of those around them by addressing the root causes of health and opportunity.

Each conversation you start, each barrier you address, each resource you share contributes to a collective journey toward a more just and caring world.

A Final Thought:

There will be days when this work feels too big, too slow, or too frustrating, and moments when progress seems invisible. In those times, remember: we do this together. You have a community and you have found support (including this toolkit).

Together: - Small steps create momentum.- Momentum leads to shifts in perspective and circumstance.- Shifts lead to transformation over time.

Every conversation, every intervention, every act of advocacy adds to the collective movement toward a more equitable world.

This is the work of social care. This is the work of change.

And it begins right here, in this moment, with you taking your next step.

CONCLUSION

You've reached the end of the Social Determinants of Health Toolkit, but in many ways, the journey is just beginning. Before we conclude, let's take a moment to reflect on what we've covered and what it means moving forward.

In reflecting on this material, I (the author) want to share some personal thoughts as we encourage you to reflect on your own experiences. Let's take a deep breath together and allow everything we've discussed to settle in.

Ask yourself:

- What is one thing I will commit to doing this week? It might be something you identified in the workbook section—a small step toward a goal.
- Who will I reach out to for support? Think of a person or group that can encourage you or help you as you work on your goals.
- How will I celebrate my progress—no matter how small? Perhaps you'll treat yourself to something you enjoy after completing a step, or simply acknowledge your effort and feel proud.

This toolkit is a guide for creating a life, a career, and a community that values well-being in every sense of the word, according to your vision for it.

No one has to do this alone. And no step is too small.

Because every action—every step toward progress, every choice to show up, every decision to create change—matters.

Reflect on the plant metaphor one more time: A plant grows strong when rooted in the right environment. It doesn't thrive because someone pours water on exposed roots; it flourishes when it's planted in rich soil—supported by everything it needs to grow. The same is true for us. No one thrives in isolation. No one overcomes challenges by simply being told to "do better" or "try harder." True transformation happens when people are given the right conditions—access to stability, education, healthcare, safe neighborhoods, strong communities, nutritious food, and meaningful work.

I encourage you (and others) to think about the following questions regularly: - Do you have someone in your life to talk about your financial security and goals for improvement?- Do you have someone you can discuss your healthcare plans and needs with?- Is there someone you trust to talk about your neighborhood—whether it feels adequate for your goals or if you have concerns about it?- Do you have someone to share your goals for continuous learning and education with?- Do you have a person with whom you feel emotionally safe discussing your social environment and how you might improve it?- Is there someone you can talk to about healthy eating goals or bringing more nutritious foods you love into your diet?- Who can you share your career or volunteer goals with—someone who can help usher in opportunities or offer guidance?

Here's the great part: if you don't have answers to some of these questions yet, you can become that person for yourself and seek out those people in your community starting today. Strengthening these "roots" in your life sustains your goals, and when they are nourished, everything above the surface—your health, your happiness, your achievements—can flourish.

This book has been an opportunity to closely examine the soil we are planted in—to look at the conditions that shape individual health and the well-being of our communities. It's been a space for reflection, a prompt to action, and an invitation to become caretakers of our own roots and stewards of the environments that sustain others. When we understand social determinants of health, we don't just see problems—we begin to see solutions. We see pathways forward, opportunities to build stronger systems, and simple ways to create meaningful change in the lives around us.

And so, the journey doesn't end here. The work continues in how we nurture our lives, advocate for those facing barriers, and empower human connections that allow everyone to take root and grow. It's about understanding that health and equity are not only medical concerns—they're deeply human concerns.

As this journey continues beyond these pages, let it be fueled by the knowledge that every action matters, no matter how small. When a barrier is acknowledged, a resource is shared, a voice is used to advocate, or a connection is strengthened, the world shifts a little. In that shift, there is hope. Because when we commit to seeing each other fully—and addressing not just the symptoms but the root causes of struggles—we move from merely imagining a better world to actively building it.

QUESTIONS

To continue your journey of reflection and growth, here is a structured set of questions you can ask yourself (or others) to assess various areas of life. These questions can help you gauge satisfaction, support, and areas for improvement across each domain of SDOH. Use them as a self-assessment tool or a conversation starter with someone you're trying to help.

Structured Social Determinants of Health Assessment Questions

Economic Stability

- How satisfied are you with your current employment situation, including job security and working conditions?
- How satisfied are you with your level of income and its stability?
- How satisfied are you with your ability to manage expenses and handle unexpected costs?
- How satisfied are you with your current level of debt (if any) and your ability to repay it?

- How satisfied are you with your ability to handle medical bills?
- How satisfied are you with the availability and quality of financial support or assistance (like public benefits or community programs)?
- To what extent do you feel you have someone you can turn to for discussing your employment situation?
- To what extent do you feel you have someone to talk to about your income stability?
- To what extent do you feel supported when discussing expenses and financial management?
- To what extent do you have a trusted person to talk to about debt management?
- To what extent do you feel you have support in discussing medical bills and healthcare costs?
- To what extent do you feel supported when seeking financial assistance or guidance?
- How would you rate the quality of safe spaces available to discuss your employment concerns?
- How would you rate the quality of safe spaces to discuss your income stability?
- How would you rate the quality of support spaces for managing expenses and budgeting?
- How would you rate the quality of spaces for discussing debt and repayment strategies?
- How would you rate the quality of spaces for discussing medical bills and related costs?

- How would you rate the quality of spaces to discuss financial support options?

Education Access and Quality

- How satisfied are you with your current access to education opportunities (formal and informal)?
- To what extent do you feel your literacy skills enable you to navigate daily tasks and professional requirements effectively?
- How would you rate the availability of language support resources (like ESL programs) in your community?
- How often do you feel supported by peers or community in pursuing educational goals?
- How accessible are vocational training programs or career development resources in your area?
- To what extent do you feel encouraged by your social circle (family, friends, mentors) to pursue personal or professional growth through education?
- How satisfied are you with the availability of early childhood education resources for your children (if applicable)?
- How confident are you in finding and accessing online educational resources (virtual courses, skill-building platforms)?
- How satisfied are you with opportunities for lifelong learning and continuing education in your community?
- How would you rate the quality of local libraries, community centers, or other public resources for educational support?

- To what extent do financial barriers limit your ability to pursue further education or training?
- How confident are you in finding mentorship or guidance to support you when you pursue educational opportunities?

Healthcare Access and Quality

- How satisfied are you with your ability to access medical care when you need it?
- How satisfied are you with the quality of healthcare services you receive?
- How satisfied are you with your ability to afford necessary healthcare services without financial stress?
- How satisfied are you with your access to mental health services and support?
- How satisfied are you with the availability of culturally competent healthcare providers in your community?
- How confident are you in navigating the healthcare system (scheduling appointments, understanding medical information, etc.)?
- How accessible are healthcare facilities, pharmacies, and emergency services from where you live?
- To what extent do you feel you have a trusted healthcare provider who understands your needs?
- To what extent do you have someone to talk to about healthcare-related decisions and concerns?
- To what extent do you feel supported when managing chronic conditions or ongoing health issues?

- How confident are you in finding reliable health information when needed?
- How satisfied are you with the availability of preventive healthcare services (vaccinations, screenings, etc.)?
- How often do you experience delays in receiving medical care due to transportation or scheduling issues?
- How satisfied are you with your ability to access affordable prescription medications?
- How confident are you in advocating for yourself when speaking with healthcare providers?
- How satisfied are you with the accessibility of healthcare options like telemedicine or mobile clinics?
- How often do you feel your healthcare concerns are taken seriously by providers?
- How would you rate your overall satisfaction with the healthcare system as it relates to your personal needs?

Neighborhood and Physical Environment

- How satisfied are you with your current housing situation (stability, affordability, condition)?
- How satisfied are you with the accessibility, affordability, and reliability of transportation options available to you?
- How satisfied are you with your neighborhood's safety and security?
- How satisfied are you with access to parks or recreational spaces in your area?

- To what extent do you feel your neighborhood fosters a sense of community and belonging?
- How satisfied are you with your neighborhood's walkability and access to essential services (stores, schools, etc.)?
- How often do you feel your geographic location limits your access to necessary resources or opportunities?
- To what extent do you have safe spaces to discuss concerns about your physical environment or housing?
- How would you rate the overall cleanliness and maintenance of your neighborhood?
- How satisfied are you with the availability of affordable housing in your area?
- How accessible are healthcare facilities or emergency services from your neighborhood?
- How often do environmental concerns (pollution, noise, extreme weather) affect your well-being?
- To what extent do you feel your neighborhood provides opportunities for social interaction and engagement?
- How satisfied are you with the availability and accessibility of grocery stores and fresh food options in your neighborhood?
- How satisfied are you with the availability of public spaces like libraries, community centers, or gathering areas?
- To what extent do you feel your neighborhood is well-lit and designed for safety at night?

- How often do you experience challenges with public utilities (clean water, electricity, waste management) in your neighborhood?
- How accessible are sidewalks and public transportation for individuals with disabilities or mobility issues?
- How satisfied are you with road conditions and infrastructure maintenance in your area?

Social and Community Context

- How satisfied are you with your ability to participate in activities with others that align with your personal interests or passions?
- How would you rate the quality of spaces available to discuss social stress or societal pressures you face?
- How satisfied are you with the quality of your current support systems (friends, family, coworkers, community)?
- How connected do you feel to your community through groups, events, or other engagement?
- What is your current stress level related to your financial status? (This ties to both economics and social perceptions.)
- To what extent do you have someone to talk to about experiences of discrimination or inequity?
- How satisfied are you with the availability of community groups, clubs, or social organizations that align with your interests?
- How often do you feel isolated or lonely, even if you have social connections?

- How confident are you in your ability to find and build new social connections if needed?
- How satisfied are you with your ability to maintain strong relationships with family and close friends?
- How often do societal expectations or pressures negatively impact your mental well-being?
- How comfortable do you feel discussing personal challenges with people in your social circle?
- How would you rate the inclusivity and diversity of the social spaces you engage in?
- How frequently do you feel heard and valued in your workplace or social environment?
- How satisfied are you with the level of emotional support you receive from those around you?
- How often do you engage in community service or volunteer activities?
- To what extent do you feel a sense of belonging in your neighborhood or city?
- How would you rate the availability of safe spaces to openly discuss personal concerns?
- How often do financial constraints limit your ability to participate in social activities?
- How confident are you in accessing local advocacy groups or organizations that support social equity and inclusion?
- How satisfied are you with your ability to resolve conflicts in your personal and professional relationships?

Food Access and Nutrition

- How satisfied are you with your ability to access healthy and quality food options?
- How satisfied are you with your access to affordable food?
- To what extent do you feel supported by friends or family in making healthy eating choices?
- How often do you feel confident in your ability to prepare healthy meals for yourself or others?
- How would you rate the availability of community resources (food grants, volunteer meal services, food banks) in your area?
- How frequently do you experience hunger or worry about having enough food?
- How satisfied are you with the variety and quality of food options in your local stores?
- How confident are you in understanding nutrition labels and making healthy food choices?
- How often do financial concerns affect your ability to buy nutritious food?
- How satisfied are you with the accessibility of grocery stores, farmers' markets, or fresh food sources nearby?
- How would you rate the availability of culturally relevant food options in your area?
- How often do you rely on fast food or highly processed meals due to convenience or affordability?
- How satisfied are you with your access to nutrition education or healthy eating programs?

- How often do you skip meals due to financial or time constraints?
- To what extent do you feel your eating habits contribute positively to your health and energy levels?
- How satisfied are you with your ability to afford and access fresh fruits and vegetables regularly?
- How often do you have difficulty getting food due to transportation issues?
- How confident are you in your ability to cook nutritious meals at home?

Work and Recreation

- How satisfied are you with your current job in terms of stability and work-life balance?
- How satisfied are you with the level of fulfillment you get from your work or professional activities?
- How satisfied are you with your ability to engage in recreational activities that bring you joy and relaxation?
- How satisfied are you with your workplace environment, including leadership support and company culture?
- How confident are you in maintaining a work-life balance without burning out?
- How accessible are opportunities for career growth and professional development in your field?
- How often do you feel your job provides you with a sense of purpose and achievement?

- To what extent do you have a supportive work environment that values your well-being?
- How satisfied are you with your ability to take breaks, time off, or vacations when needed?
- To what extent do you have access to recreational spaces, fitness centers, or outdoor areas for exercise and leisure?
- How satisfied are you with your ability to pursue hobbies and personal interests outside of work?
- To what extent do financial concerns limit your ability to participate in recreational activities?
- How confident are you in setting boundaries between work time and personal time?
- How often do you feel socially connected with coworkers or professional peers?
- How satisfied are you with the availability of work benefits such as paid leave, wellness programs, or flexible work arrangements?
- How often do you experience stress related to work obligations?
- How satisfied are you with your access to career counseling, mentorship, or networking opportunities?
- How would you rate the overall quality of your work and recreation balance in life?

These questions can guide your reflection or be used as part of a structured assessment (perhaps in a journal or with a counselor). Answer them honestly for yourself to identify areas of strength and areas that might need attention or support.

They can also be revisited over time to gauge improvement or changes in your circumstances and perceptions.

By continually considering these questions, you maintain awareness of how different aspects of your life are affecting your health and happiness. They help ensure that as life changes, you adjust and seek support where needed. Remember, the goal is not to achieve a "perfect" score in every category, but to be mindful of how these factors interplay and to strive for improvement and support where you can.

RESOURCES AND APPENDICES

In this section, you'll find a compilation of resources, data sources, and practical tools to further support you. Whether you're looking for evidence-based research, practical guides, or community programs, these are meant to serve as a "toolbox" you can draw from as needed.

Data Sources and Research on Social Determinants of Health

For evidence-based insights and real-world applications of SDOH, consider exploring the following:

- **Healthy People 2030** (**U.S. Department of Health & Human Services**) - Comprehensive goals and objectives related to SDOH, tracking national progress in key areas. (Website: health.gov/healthypeople)
- **Centers for Disease Control and Prevention** (**CDC**) - **SDOH Data & Statistics** - Extensive reports and interactive data tools examining health disparities and social determinants at local, state, and national levels. (Website: cdc.gov/socialdeterminants)
- **World Health Organization** (**WHO**) - **Commission on Social Determinants of Health** - Global

perspectives and policy recommendations for addressing SDOH. (Website: who.int/social_determinants)

- **Kaiser Family Foundation (KFF) – SDOH and Health Equity Research** – Analysis of Medicaid, Medicare, and other approaches to integrating SDOH into healthcare policies. (Website: kff.org)
- **National Alliance to Impact the Social Determinants of Health (NASDOH) Reports** – Coalition-based insights on cross-sector collaboration improving SDOH outcomes. (Website: nasdoh.org)
- **National Association of Community Health Workers (NACHW) Case Studies** – Real-world examples of CHWs addressing SDOH through community initiatives. (Website: nachw.org)

These sources provide in-depth data, case studies, and policy recommendations if you wish to dive deeper into the topic or need credible information for advocacy and programming.

Practical Tools for Implementing SDOH Strategies

These resources offer actionable templates and guides for integrating SDOH into your work or personal life:

- **SDOH Assessment and Screening Tools:** - PRAPARE (Protocol for Responding to and Assessing Patients' Assets, Risks, and Experiences) – A standardized screening tool used in clinics and community settings to assess patients' social needs. (Download via National Association of Community

Health Centers (NACHC) - search for PRAPARE Toolkit)

- **Social Needs Screening & Referral Tool** (**Aunt Bertha/FindHelp**) - A digital platform to connect individuals to local services based on assessed needs.(Website: findhelp.org)

Goal-Setting and Action Plan Templates: - Personal SDOH Roadmap Template - A guided worksheet (much like the one we did in the workbook section) to help individuals identify priority SDOH areas, set measurable goals, and track progress. (Try creating your own based on the workbook prompts, or search for "SDOH personal action plan template".)

- **Community Intervention Planning Guide** - If you're a professional developing local SDOH initiatives, look for step-by-step guides or toolkits from organizations like the Build Healthy Places Network or ChangeLab Solutions that provide frameworks for creating community-level change.

Advocacy and Policy Resources:

- **National Academy of Medicine** (**NAM**)
- **SDOH Policy Recommendations**

Research-backed policy briefs and recommendations for integrating SDOH into public health and healthcare. (Website: nam.edu, search SDOH projects.)

- **Public Health Law Center - SDOH and Legal Advocacy** - Resources on using policy and law to address structural inequalities in healthcare and social services. (Website: publichealthlawcenter.org)

- **Community Advocacy Toolkit (ChangeLab Solutions)** – Practical guidance on mobilizing local communities for policy change tailored to SDOH issues. (Website: changelabsolutions.org)

Funding Opportunities for SDOH Initiatives: - Robert Wood Johnson Foundation (RWJF) Grants – This foundation often funds projects aimed at health equity and SDOH. (Website: rwjf.org)

- **Health Resources & Services Administration (HRSA) – SDOH-Focused Grants** – Federal grants supporting community health initiatives, especially in underserved areas. (Website: hrsa.gov/grants, look for grants related to health equity or community health.)
- **Grantmakers In Health (GIH) – Social Impact Funding Database** – A resource to find philanthropic and government funding sources for SDOH projects. (Website: gih.org)

Training and Continuing Education on SDOH: - CDC TRAIN – Free SDOH Training Courses – Online modules for healthcare providers, social workers, and public health professionals on SDOH. (Website: train.org/cdctrain)

- **American Public Health Association (APHA) – SDOH Certificate Program** – Specialized training in policy, community organizing, and health equity. (Website: APHA.org, search for continuing education or certificates.)
- **Harvard Online Course: Improving Health Outcomes through SDOH** – A case-based learning experience teaching strategies to integrate SDOH

considerations into practice. (Website: Harvard's online platform or search for Harvard SDOH course.)

Additional Resources for Enhancing Each of the Seven SDOH Areas

The following are practical, user-friendly resources that emphasize real-world application, community support, and self-empowerment. They're categorized by SDOH area:

Economic Stability – Financial Literacy and Employment Support: - MyMoney.gov – A government-run financial literacy site with budgeting tools, savings guides, and debt management tips. (Website: mymoney.gov)

- **National Foundation for Credit Counseling** (**NFCC**) – Offers free/low-cost financial counseling, including debt relief and budgeting workshops. (Website: nfcc.org)
- **CareerOneStop** (**U.S. Department of Labor**) – Provides job training programs, career exploration tools, and workforce support. (Website: careeronestop.org)
- **211.org** (**United Way**) – A nationwide resource hotline and website connecting people to local financial assistance, job training, emergency resources, etc. (Website: 211.org or just dial 2-1-1.)
- **LinkedIn Learning Free Courses** – Occasionally offers free professional development courses on resume building, networking, and skills (access via public libraries or promotions). (Website: linkedin.com/learning)

Neighborhood and Built Environment – Housing and Transportation: - National Low Income Housing Coalition – Resources on affordable housing programs, tenant rights, and rental assistance. (Website: nlihc.org)

- **LIHEAP (Low-Income Home Energy Assistance Program**) – Helps low-income families with energy costs, weatherization, and utility bills. (Website: acf.hhs.gov/ocs/liheap)
- **Ride United (United Way & Lyft partnership**) – Provides free or low-cost rides for medical appointments, grocery trips, job interviews in certain areas. (Website: check unitedway.org for Ride United info.)
- **National Volunteer Transportation Center** – Connects individuals with community-based volunteer ride services (good for elderly or disabled). (Website: nationalvolunteertransportationcenter.org)
- **Safe Routes to School** (**SRTS**) – Program to improve walkability and biking for children, enhancing neighborhood safety for students. (Website: saferoutesinfo.org)
- **EPA Environmental Justice Grant**s – Funding and resources to address environmental hazards in low-income areas (useful if your community faces pollution issues). (Website: epa.gov/environmentaljustice)

Education Access and Quality – Learning Resources and Support: - Khan Academy – Free educational courses from basic math and reading to advanced subjects, great for all ages. (Website: khanacademy.org)

- **Coursera & edX Free Courses** – University-level courses from institutions like Harvard, MIT, etc., often free to audit. (Websites: coursera.org and edx.org)
- **GED Testing Service** – Resources for adults seeking a high school equivalency diploma, including study guides and test info. (Website: ged.com)
- **ProLiteracy** – A network of adult literacy programs offering reading, writing, and workforce skills education. (Website: proliteracy.org)
- **Understood.org** – Resource hub for parents and educators supporting children with learning differences (ADHD, dyslexia, etc.). (Website: understood.org)
- **College Board BigFuture** – Scholarship searches, college planning, and financial aid guidance for students. (Website: bigfuture.collegeboard.org)

Food Security and Nutrition – Access and Healthy Eating: - Feeding America – A national network of food banks providing free meals and produce; find your local food bank. (Website: feedingamerica.org)

- **Meals on Wheels** – Delivers healthy meals to older adults and those with disabilities nationwide. (Website: mealsonwheelsamerica.org)
- **ChooseMyPlate (USDA)** – Offers personalized nutrition guidance and meal-planning resources in an easy visual format. (Website: choosemyplate.gov)
- **Budget Bytes** – A website featuring healthy, budget-friendly recipes with cost per meal calculated. Great

for stretching food dollars. (Website: budgetbytes.com)

Social and Community Context – Social Support and Engagement: - Meetup.com – Helps individuals find and join local social groups based on common interests (from hiking to book clubs to tech meetups). (Website: meetup.com)

- **National Alliance on Mental Illness (NAMI) Support Groups** – Free peer support groups for individuals and families dealing with mental health challenges, available nationwide. (Website: nami.org, look for local support groups.)
- **VolunteerMatch** – Connects people with volunteer opportunities aligned with their skills and passions (great for meeting people and giving back). (Website: volunteermatch.org)
- **AmeriCorps** – Opportunities to serve communities across the U.S. while gaining skills and possibly education benefits. (Website: americorps.gov)

Healthcare Access and Quality – Finding Affordable Care and Support: - HRSA Health Centers (Health Resources & Services Administration) – Federally funded clinics offering medical, dental, and mental health care on a sliding scale (no one turned away for inability to pay). (Find one near you: findahealthcenter.hrsa.gov)

- **Telehealth.HHS.gov** – Government guide to finding low-cost or free telehealth services, improving remote healthcare access. (Website: telehealth.hhs.gov)
- **988 Suicide & Crisis Lifeline** – Free, confidential crisis support 24/7 via phone or text for mental

health emergencies. (Just dial or text 988, Website: 988lifeline.org)

- **Mental Health America (MHA) Screening Tool** - Free, anonymous online mental health screenings for conditions like depression or anxiety, with guidance on next steps. (Website: mhascreening.org)
- **NeedyMeds** - A resource for finding assistance with medication costs, clinic locations, and even medical transportation options. (Website: needymeds.org)
- **Patient Advocate Foundation** - Helps patients navigate healthcare bureaucracy (insurance issues, billing, etc.) and can connect to financial aid programs. (Website: patientadvocate.org)

Final Thoughts on Utilizing These Resources

These tools, services, and organizations are stepping stones toward greater well-being. Whether your goal is securing financial stability, improving access to education, strengthening your social support, or advocating for better healthcare, each resource offers a tangible way to move forward. The key to lasting progress is taking small, intentional steps and using the right support systems to turn knowledge into action.

Keep this "toolbox" handy. You don't need every tool all the time, but it's good to know they're there. And remember: reaching out for resources or help is a sign of strength, not weakness.

Your voice and efforts make an incredible difference. By leveraging resources and staying committed, you help shape a healthier, more equitable future—for yourself, those around you, and your broader community.

Your Voice Makes an Incredible Difference: Help Shape the Future of Healthcare

(A note from the author and team behind this toolkit:)

We're grateful that you've taken the time to journey through this book to the very end. This shows your commitment to understanding and improving health through social determinants, and we want to invite you to be part of spreading the word.

It might surprise you, but roughly 85% of readers are more likely to purchase a book when they see a strong collection of thoughtful reviews. Your review isn't just feedback for us or information for other readers—it's a catalyst that helps more people discover and benefit from the insights in these pages.

If this toolkit offered you valuable knowledge, challenged your perspective, or equipped you with tools to make a difference, we'd be honored if you'd take a minute to share your thoughts in a review.

Every review expands our reach, ensuring that more healthcare leaders, educators, community members, and changemakers can join in re-humanizing healthcare through a deeper understanding of social determinants of health.

How to Leave a Review (Quick Steps): 1. Use your phone's camera to scan the QR code below (or search for the book's title on Amazon or your bookseller's site).2. The link will take you to the review page.3. Share your rating and a brief review.

(If the QR code or direct link doesn't work for your location, you can use the link in your order confirmation email or simply navigate to the book's page on the site and click "Leave a Review.")

Taking just 60 seconds to do this makes a world of difference. Thank you for being part of this mission. Your support fuels the impact of this work. Together, we are shaping a healthier, more equitable world.

ADDITIONAL SERVICES

As we conclude, we want to let you know about some additional services and opportunities available through Dr. Jeremy Holloway (the author) and the Tellegacy organization that produced this toolkit. These services are designed to help you unlock the power of intergenerational connection, transformative leadership, and practical social care solutions in your community or organization.

Tellegacy: Bridging Generations, Strengthening Communities

The Tellegacy Intergenerational Program is a nationally recognized initiative designed to reduce social isolation, enhance well-being, and build meaningful connections between older adults and students. It's rooted in evidence-based practices and is helping healthcare organizations, universities, and communities cultivate engagement that improves behavioral health outcomes.

Through Tellegacy, we: - Implement intergenerational programs in healthcare systems, academic institutions, and community organizations.- Provide structured training and resources to ensure these programs integrate seamlessly and effectively.- Foster a movement that strengthens both older and younger generations through shared experiences.

Learn More or Bring Tellegacy to Your Organization: Visit tellegacy.org for more information, case studies, and contact details if you're interested in launching Tellegacy programs in your setting.

Keynote Speaking & Leadership Engagements

Dr. Jeremy Holloway is also a national speaker, educator, and thought leader in health equity, intergenerational innovation, and workforce development. His presentations challenge conventional thinking and inspire real change across sectors - from healthcare to education to nonprofit leadership.

Dr. Holloway's keynotes and workshops often focus on: - Health equity and social determinants of health (making the case for why addressing SDOH is urgent and how to do it effectively).- Intergenerational strategies to reduce social isolation (sharing the Tellegacy model and outcomes).- Behavioral health and combating loneliness (especially relevant for aging populations or during times like the pandemic).- Leadership and workforce development in healthcare (how to cultivate an empathetic, forward-thinking workforce).

Whether it's for a national conference, an industry summit, or an organization's leadership retreat, these sessions are designed to inform, engage, and transform perspectives - leaving audiences with actionable insights.

Interested in Booking Dr. Holloway? Visit jeremyholloway.com/speaker/ for speaking topics, testimonials, and booking inquiries.

Consulting for Healthcare & Nonprofits

For organizations looking to enhance their impact on social determinants or integrate intergenerational and equity-focused programs, Dr. Holloway offers strategic consulting services:

Areas of consulting expertise include: - Implementing health equity and intergenerational programs (like Tellegacy or other community health initiatives).- Workforce development and leadership training with a focus on empathy, social care, and innovation.- Community engagement strategies that bridge healthcare with social services and education.- Behavioral health strategies aimed at improving patient and staff outcomes (addressing issues like burnout, mental health, and social support networks).

With deep experience in program development, training, and on-the-ground implementation, Dr. Holloway partners with organizations to create sustainable solutions that drive measurable change.

Interested in Consultation? Visit jeremyholloway.com/consulting/ to learn more and schedule an exploratory call.

Take the Next Step with Us

If this toolkit resonated with you and you're looking to expand its impact: - Integrate Tellegacy into your healthcare or education system to connect generations and improve well-being. - Engage Dr. Holloway for a keynote or workshop to ignite passion and understanding around SDOH and social care in your team or community. - Strengthen your organization with custom consulting solutions that help turn these principles into practice.

For more information or to get in touch: - Visit tellegacy.org for program details and additional resources. - Inquire about speaking or consulting via tellegacy.org/contact or the contact form on Dr. Holloway's website.

Building a healthier, more connected world starts with leadership, strategy, and action. We're excited to work together to make it happen.

Thank you for reading, learning, and taking action. Here's to the work ahead and the brighter futures we are creating, one step at a time.

www.ingramcontent.com/pod-product-compliance
Lightning Source LLC
LaVergne TN
LVHW050822061126
851857LV00012B/926
9798182718882